Working with Dangerous People
The psychotherapy of violence

Edited by

David Jones

Psychoanalytic Psychotherapist
Therapist, Assessment Unit
Grendon Prison
United Kingdom

Forewords by

Christopher Cordess

Psychoanalyst
Emeritus Professor of Forensic Psychiatry
University of Sheffield

and

Terry A Kupers

Psychiatrist
Institute Professor
The Wright Institute
Berkeley, California

RADCLIFFE MEDICAL PRESS

OXFORD • SAN FRANCISCO

Radcliffe Medical Press Ltd
18 Marcham Road
Abingdon
Oxon OX14 1AA
United Kingdom

www.radcliffe-oxford.com
The Radcliffe Medical Press electronic catalogue and online ordering facility.
Direct sales to anywhere in the world.

British Library Cataloguing in Publication Data

A catalogue record for this book is available from the British Library.

ISBN 1 85775 824 2

Typeset by Anne Joshua & Associates, Oxford
Printed and bound in Great Britain by TJI Digital, Padstow, Cornwall

Contents

Foreword

It is an honour to be asked to write a foreword to this admirable volume which is in so many ways close to my heart in conception and content.

Contemporary policy responses to increasing violence and a perception of an increasing prevalence of dangerous people tend towards the increasingly coercive and authoritarian; for example, escalations of surveillance, expanding legislation and a mushrooming of the size of the prison population. We have, indeed, in recent decades in Western societies, moved from a 'Culture of Welfare' to a 'Culture of Control'.[1] Many of us working within the health and welfare systems related to the criminal justice system consider these policies to be barren, especially when they ignore or neglect the complex but crucial issues of institutional and prison culture, treatment and rehabilitation. Professionals working in these fields increasingly feel over-regulated and restricted by policies in which they, working at the coal face, frequently have little faith. Add to this the anxieties for the clinician of being held responsible – within the culture of blame – for even the least predictable of his client's actions, and we have the ingredients for a dangerously de-moralised system.

This book, written by people with an intimate knowledge of prisons and dangerous prisoners and their mental health and welfare, offers something of an antidote to the simply coercive and repressive. In the words of the editor, it offers 'a humane approach to working with dangerous people . . . It should be a basic tenet of psychological work with clients that we are prepared and able to be in sympathy with them, to have some understanding of their despair'. The rich source of knowledge and experience of the contributors is that gleaned largely from working at, or in close association with, the therapeutic community at Grendon Underwood Prison; the contents have wide and far reaching applicability to all aspects of understanding the anti-social and dangerous offender.

Forensic psychotherapy – the attempted amelioration of psychological pathology and criminal behaviour in the criminal offender – always operates within a triangulated system in which society, represented by its institutions (e.g. the criminal justice system), has a legitimate and important role, in addition to the therapist and client dyad.

Actually, as our society becomes more and more preoccupied with risk assessment and risk management, and third party protection, society's concerns impinge upon all psychotherapy, even that which appears most 'private and voluntary' – but that is another subject. Psychotherapy, by its nature, questions the premises upon which beliefs, whether individual, institutional or societal, are held. Such a questioning is at the heart of the operation of the therapeutic community. It is a highly commendable feature of this book that it encourages examination and re-examination of assumptions too easily made and taken for granted. So that, whereas it is primarily concerned with 'the mind of the criminal' (and his behaviour) it also takes cognizance of 'the criminal of the mind', that is to say those aspects of ourselves which are potentially anti-social, criminal or neglectful. In this context, this may be focused down to the potential for abusive or excessively retaliatory policies or individual behaviour, and in settings of detention the ever present tendencies towards quite subtle, as well as gross, abuses of power. Our 'criminal institutions' are every bit in need of assessment and 'treatment' as the dangerous people held within them, but they are frequently even more resistant.

Theory – implicit or explicit – and practice are intimately entwined in all good psychotherapy, as indeed in any criminological endeavour. For heuristic reasons, as has become traditional, this book is divided into separate theory and practice parts, but it seems to me that they are especially well integrated. I particularly enjoyed the philosophically well informed critique by Agnes Petocz of 'scientism' in psychology and the way in which the 'evidence based' movement has been applied in a form which is often a concretised caricature of its progenitor's original intention. Clearly and relatedly, it is of crucial importance in our subject that we fully participate in the contemporary rapprochement between the neurosciences and the 'psychotherapies of meaning', rather than allow ourselves to become caught up in furthering that false divide.

This volume offers a contribution to ways of thinking about dangerous people and their behaviour, and working with them constructively, respectfully and possibly redemptively.

Although there is no chapter dedicated to the subject of training, supervision and professional support, these crucial aspects are implicit, and sometimes explicit, throughout the text. I sincerely hope that this book will be read by all those concerned with offenders in whatever capacity, from clinicians to politicians, from policy makers to managers. It will well reward their interest and attention.

Christopher Cordess
Psychoanalyst
Emeritus Professor of Forensic Psychiatry
University of Sheffield
January 2004

Reference

1   Garland D (2001) *The Culture of Control.* Oxford University Press, Oxford.

Foreword

I don't believe it is overly optimistic to say we are witnessing the beginning of a paradigm shift in the field of criminology. The reigning paradigm, the one that is about to be replaced, involves an ever more punitive approach to criminal defendants and prisoners. Punish, punish, punish: less sympathy in the courts, longer sentences, fewer privileges behind bars, less recourse, tougher parole officers, more parole violations, added prison time. The singularly punitive approach has had its trial, and, in the minds of many policy-makers and correctional managers, it has proven a failure. In the period that began with Robert Martinson's[1] 1974 'nothing works' proclamation about efforts at rehabilitation, rehab programs have been dismantled, the prisons have become massively overcrowded, and harsher punishments have been instituted at every turn. Meanwhile there is more violence in the prisons, the crime rate in the community did not fall, but the recidivism rate rose, as did the proportion of prisoners serving time merely for violating parole. The punitive approach does not help dangerous people take control of their aggressive impulses. Today, the big question is, if ever harsher punishments don't work, what will? Specifically, what is the most effective intervention with the disruptive and assaultive prisoner?

The story of supermaximum security prisons in the USA is emblematic of the evolving paradigm shift. Supermaxes (also known as maxi-maxis, control units, security housing units or SHUs) exploded on the corrections scene a little over a decade ago. The idea was to curtail the frighteningly high rate of prison violence by locking assaultive prisoners in their concrete and steel cells most of 24 hours per day. Of course, there was a certain quieting of the prison yards for a while, the quarantine effect. But beyond the immediate quieting, the outcome is not as cheering. For example, there is the problem of 'maxing out of the SHU'. So many prisoners are relegated to long-term isolated confinement that a certain number of them reach their fixed release date prior to finishing their stint in the SHU. They are released into the community straight out of a cell where they had been isolated and idle for years. Not surprisingly, some of them return to drugs and alcohol and commit heinous crimes. What is surprising is that there aren't more who do so. Most ex-inhabitants of supermaximum isolation cells actually keep to themselves when they are released from prison, their will to relate to others having been broken. But when any ex-resident of supermax commits a violent crime there are headlines and, of course, heated accusations about where the fault lies.

The 'tough on crime' faction loudly proclaim that the heinous deed is incontrovertible proof the violent criminal element is incorrigible, and call for a halt to 'coddling' and the building of even more super-secure prisons where we can 'lock-'em-up-and-throw-away-the-key'. The other side in the debate, prison reformers and progressives among them, just as passionately believe that the error was to lock prisoners in cold storage in the first place; long-term isolated confinement causes human breakdown of all kinds, including psychosis, suicide, and in far too many cases, intensification of uncontrollable violent impulses. To the reformers, the crime spree of an ex-SHU resident means that the corrections department has failed in its mission to reduce violence and 'correct' the errant felon. After all, the first principle of interventions aimed at reducing violence is to make certain that the interventions themselves do not actually raise the prevalence of violence; and many commentators are coming to the conclusion that the advent of the supermaximum security prison has increased rather than decreased the rates of violence in the prisons and on the streets.

Of course, both sides in this very old debate haul out scientific studies to bolster their arguments. Often, the two sides utilize the same events and the same statistics to make very opposite points. An example is the fact that people who have committed violent acts in the past are more likely than others to commit violent acts in the future. This well-known correlation can be used to buffet the argument that they must be locked up for a very long time and punished severely, or the same correlation can be used to support the argument that we need to find programs that work to change the deeply ingrained habits of very assaultive individuals or else we will suffer the consequences of their repeated acts of violence after they are released from custody.

Clearly, anyone who steps forward to proclaim a new, less exclusively punitive paradigm for corrections must first argue that there is scientific evidence for their approach, that the arguments of their 'tough on crime' adversaries have indeed proven a failure, and that the interventions and programs being proposed are effective in managing and rehabilitating assaultive prisoners. If the crime rate has not fallen substantially in the face of the unprecedented imprisonment binge in the USA in recent decades, then it is not going to be possible to prevent violent crime by locking up an even greater proportion of the population. And even political conservatives are realizing the practical folly of a strategy that relies on ever tougher sentencing: it costs a lot of money to keep so many people in prison, and even with today's harsher penalties, most prisoners will eventually be released. Do we want them to come out of prison broken and embittered by the constant punishments, and by the many cruelties that inevitably evolve within a culture of punishment? Meanwhile, class action lawsuits are forcing the states and the federal government to pay more respect to human and civil rights, and that means halting the kinds of abuse that regularly crop up in the extremity of supermaximum confinement. The tide is turning and a growing number of serious criminologists and policy-makers are asking what alternatives there might be to ever longer prison sentences. The state of Maryland has announced it will close its supermaximum facility near Baltimore, and other states are thinking about following suit.

But there is a problem. The staff will have to talk to the prisoners. Too often in the supermax setting the officers limit their contact with prisoners to barking out orders and cussing them as they tell them what will happen to them if they deign to disobey. In the highly segregated and controlled setting that the modern maximum security prison has become, many staff have forgotten how to talk civilly to a prisoner, how to ask a prisoner how he is feeling and what are his needs, and how to interact casually with prisoners on the yard or in the dayroom. One can see the result in almost any maximum security prison: officers huddled in an office while the prisoners steer clear of them for fear of being labeled a 'snitch' by their peers if they engage staff in anything other than brusque exchanges.

As the paradigm shifts from punitive idleness and isolation to an emphasis on educational and rehabilitative programs, the staff must learn anew to mingle with prisoners. How will they remain safe doing their work? Which attitudes and approaches toward prisoners are most conducive to rehabilitative efforts, especially when the prisoner has a history of violence? In the old days staff interacted with rowdy prisoners on the maximum security yards. But many corrections officers and correctional mental health staff have forgotten how to do that.

By the time a scientific paradigm actually shifts, the founders of the next and better explanatory theory stand in the wings, ready to point the way forward. When Heisenberg's uncertainty principle replaced Newton's model, the group of quantum physicists at work on the new paradigm was already very sophisticated.

During the heyday of the punishment paradigm and the supermaximum prison, the staff at Grendon Prison were experimenting with a very different strategy for managing and rehabilitating assaultive prisoners. This book is both a collection of essays about their sophisticated, pioneering approach, and a preview of the new paradigm. Authors of the very varied but always thoughtful chapters about different aspects of work with very dangerous people share in common the conviction that mutual respect between ward and warder is a cardinal prerequisite for altering the behavior of disruptive and assaultive prisoners. The authors share a preference for horizontal communications over strictly top-down ones, and thus they view the prisoner as a very active participant in decisions that affect him or her. The authors prefer collaborative analysis of the meaning of events to shouting orders. And the authors deeply ascribe to the principle that more and better communication between staff and prisoners is required if we are to accomplish any significant work with very disruptive prisoners.

Grendon Prison has a unique history. As prison managements elsewhere in the United Kingdom and the USA turned to intensified segregation as the antidote to uncontrollable prisons, the staff at Grendon remained true to their plan to run a prison unit for very assaultive prisoners as a therapeutic community. Groups become the place to talk about the meaning of angry feelings, and there is significant evidence that the approach works, for example there is far less physical violence at Grendon than at other prisons of comparable security level. The editor has brought together in this eloquent volume the ideas of various participants in the Grendon experiment, along with others who have been thinking along similar lines.

And the authors have done something quite admirable: they have reintroduced psychoanalytic concepts into the field of forensic mental health – but not in the idealistic way that August Aichhorn,[2] Franz Alexander[3] and Erich Fromm[4] did early in the Twentieth Century. Rather, they have incorporated psychoanalytic or psychodynamic concepts into a growing body of theory about working with prisoners. They do not fall into the facile argument that psychoanalysis is better than cognitive behavior therapy (CBT) or any other method for prisoners who have trouble managing their tempers – they are fully aware of research findings that psychodynamic interventions by themselves are not very helpful. So they weave together our accumulated understanding of what works, they integrate diverse strategies, and they include sufficient philosophy of science to make the argument that their approach is rooted in scientific method and that it is effective. Readers will be inspired and delighted as I was to read here about the much-needed new paradigm in corrections.

Terry A Kupers MD, MSP
Institute Professor
The Wright Institute
Berkeley, California
January 2004

References

1 Martinson R (1974) What Works? Questions and answers about prison reform. *The Public Interest.* **10**: 22–54.
2 Aichhorn A (1984) *Wayward Youth.* Northwestern University Press. Originally published in the 1920s.
3 Alexander F and Staub H (1965) *The Criminal, the Judge and the Public.* The Free Press, New York. Originally published in the 1930s.
4 Fro Andersson K (1998) The young Erich Fromm's contribution to criminology. *Justice Quarterly.* **15**(4): 667–96.

List of contributors

Catherine Appleton BA, MPhil has been a research officer at the Centre for Criminological Research, University of Oxford, since 1998. Since joining the Centre she has worked on a number of different projects in the areas of youth justice, prison and probation. Most recently she has been working on a project investigating the role of the probation service in the management and resettlement of discretionary life-sentenced offenders.

Jane Coltman is a prison officer who has had a varied life as a mother, car assembly worker and mature student. For the past three years she has worked as a facilitator of one of the groups at Grendon.

Andrew Downie is the therapist for a therapeutic community of 40 prisoners, one of the five communities plus an induction assessment unit that constitute HMP Grendon. He has been in post for five and a half years. Having previously worked for a number of years as a probation officer, he trained as a group analytic psychotherapist, and chose to continue to specialise in forensic work.

Jinnie Jeffries is a psychodramatist and counselling psychologist at HMP Grendon. She has worked extensively across the world and written a number of papers and chapters.

David Jones initially took Social Studies and then trained as a social worker in psychiatry. He worked in his first therapeutic community in 1974 and then in various psychiatric and group settings in London and Oxford. He trained as a psychoanalytic psychotherapist in 1985 and then worked in a General Practice, with political refugees and running a counselling service in Oxford-shire. He entered the Prison Service in 2000 and now leads the assessment unit at Grendon Prison.

Liz McLure RMN, RGN is a group analyst, is double trained in nursing and has worked in many mental health settings. She is a qualified group analyst and works as a sessional psychotherapist at Grendon Prison.

Mark Morris trained as a doctor, psychiatrist and psychoanalyst. He worked at the Cassel Hospital in London and was then Director of Therapy at Grendon Prison. He now works at the Portman Clinic in London.

Michael Parker is currently Director of Therapy at HMP Winchester, West Hill, the first women's democratic therapeutic community prison. Before this he was at HMP Grendon, where he worked on accrediting the democratic therapeutic community method, which was incorporated within the Prison Service What Works Strategy. He is qualified as a group analyst.

Agnes Petocz is a senior lecturer in the psychology department at the University of Western Sydney. She teaches courses in the history and philosophy of psychology, personality theory, psycholinguistics and critical thinking. Her research interests include symbolism, the philosophy of psycho-analysis, the tensions between qualitative and quantitative research perspectives and the place of the concept of meaning within realist, scientific psychology. She is the author of *Freud, Psychoanalysis and Symbolism* (1999, CUP).

Gillian Proctor is a clinical psychologist working in Yorkshire, UK. She uses the person-centred approach in all aspects of her work in forensic services in the National Health Service. Her particular interests are power, ethics and oppression in relation to clinical practice, mental health systems and research. She has authored several articles on these subjects and her book *The Dynamics of Power in Counselling and Psychotherapy: ethics, politics and practice* was published by PCCS Books in 2002.

Richard Shuker is a chartered forensic psychologist and Head of Psychology at HMP Grendon. He has managed cognitive behavioural programmes within a therapeutic community for personality-disordered offenders and previously worked with young offenders. His special interest is in needs assessment and treatment of high risk offenders.

Celia Taylor trained as a forensic psychiatrist at the Institute of Psychiatry, London, and has experience in working in a variety of forensic services, from maximum secure to the community. For the last five years she has run a specialist medium secure unit for the assessment and treatment of per-sonality-disordered patients, and has become particularly interested in the effects these individuals have upon staff, institutions and relationships between professionals. She now works at the John Howard Centre, London.

Hans Toch is Distinguished Professor at the School of Criminal Justice, University at Albany, State University of New York in the USA. He holds a PhD in psychology from Princeton University. He has published extensively. His most recent books are *Acting Out: maladaptive behavior in confinement* (2002) (with Ken Adams, American Psychological Association) and *Stress in Policing* (2003, American Psychological Association).

A mad animal
Man's a mad animal
I'm a thousand years old and in my time
I've helped commit a million murders
The earth is spread
The earth is spread thick
With squashed human guts

Peter Weiss, *Marat Sade* – 1964

On the pavement
of my trampled soul
the soles of madmen
stamp the prints of crude, rude words.

Vladimir Mayakovsky, *I* – 1912

All men dream, but not equally. Those who dream by night, in the dusty recesses of their minds, awake in the day to find that it was vanity. But the dreamers of the day are dangerous men, for they may act their dreams with open eyes to make it reality.

TE Lawrence

Introduction

David Jones

Controversial issues

There is deliberate irony in the title of this book since the label 'dangerous people' gives us the opportunity, should we want it, of ignoring the individuality of our subjects and dealing with them simply as troublesome objects to be kept secure. There is no doubt that our subjects are dangerous in certain circumstances and yet in our work we discover the frightened, vulnerable, immature parts of them. To quote a colleague, Joseph Marr, they are big hairy babies. But babies would be dangerous too if they had the muscle development to carry out their impulses. It should be a basic tenet of psychological work with clients that we are prepared and able to be in sympathy with them, to have some understanding of their despair.

Many of the events described in this book will fill us with horror and despair. They have crossed the boundaries of acceptable behaviour by a considerable distance and left dozens of ruined lives in their wake. It is understandable that ordinary people reading of these in their daily newspapers or hearing the gory details described on the television would wish for their world to be made safe from the possibility of murder, rape or robbery. For these are the crimes committed by the (mainly) men who people the pages of this book.

It is perhaps only to be expected that where such passionate, dramatic and painful matters are concerned there will be controversy. And so it is. Controversy abounds in areas of social policy, psychiatric definition, potential for and appropriateness of treatment. There are powerful lobby groups representing different treatment schools. Increasingly, psychological therapies are being manualised and sold for profit and this has an impact on availability of information and the quality of academic debate. This book certainly looks at these issues. But more than that, in these pages you will find chapters describing therapeutic work in exquisite detail and offering hope that offenders can be treated humanely and effectively. Not that this is easy. There are many obstacles to successful treatment, including social and genetic factors, impatient administrators and politicians and deeply entrenched personality features. Even managing a tolerant, therapeutically oriented setting can be difficult and wearing for staff because of the attritional nature of these relationships and the inevitable boundary-pushing which raises the anxiety of all, but particularly outside observers.

Why do we keep these men in prison and attempt to help them change? Consider the alternative. In the United States the death penalty has been allowed since 1976. Research has identified that election-year political considerations may play a role in determining the timing of executions. This shows that states are approximately 25% more likely to conduct executions in gubernatorial election years than in other years. The researchers also found that elections have a larger effect on the probability that an African-American defendant will be executed in a given year than on the probability that a white defendant will be executed, and that the overall effect of elections is largest in the South.[1] If you are black then your chances of being executed are dramatically higher.[2] Then there are the innocent, of whom over a hundred have been released from death row. Although this may seem like a vindication of the justice system, it is only those who have been able to afford the best legal assistance or enlist the aid of powerful media who stand a chance of release.

The United States stands with China and Iran as among the highest users of the death penalty.

In the United Kingdom the situation is rather different. There is little possibility of the reintroduction of the death penalty but concern does exist about the disposal of men who commit such serious crimes. In particular, the Home Secretary is keen to see lifer tariffs (the term of imprisonment given to serve justice and retribution) increased to actual life for sadistic killers, 30 years for a second category including killers of policemen and prison officers, and 15 years for others. These are large increases and could have serious implications for prison numbers and for good order. The longer a prisoner's sentence is, the less is the incentive to behave well or to change for the better.

The second controversial development in the United Kingdom is the introduction of a legal and therapeutic structure for those people designated as having a Dangerous and Severe Personality Disorder (DSPD). The term 'DSPD' is not a diagnosis. It is a working title used to describe a programme of work to develop better ways of managing the relatively small number of people with a severe personality disorder who, because of their disorder, also pose a significant risk of serious harm to others. This is the description offered by the Home Office. Another way of looking at it is that so great is the concern about a small group of men that this is an attempt to take them out, to remove them from proximity with the general public, some before they have committed an offence that would make them liable to imprisonment. Alongside this statutory process there is a fairly determined effort to plan to manage them and to provide treatment to reduce the risk that they pose. The current thinking suggests that the therapeutic community model currently has the most promising evidence base in an area where the research base is rather thin.[3]

Which treatment? What is treatment?

For most people who work in the field of forensic psychotherapy it clear that the work is very difficult and that it is unworthy to make extravagant claims of success, particularly when they are made at the expense of colleagues. As Christopher Cordess states at the beginning of his seminal work ' . . . forensic psychotherapy always implies a corporate endeavour'.[4] This implies a multi-disciplinary team, usually containing psychiatrists, nurses or prison officers, psychologists, psychotherapists together with the skills of a wide range of other practitioners. It is strange therefore that within prison and correctional services in North America and the United Kingdom a virtual monoculture exists. The nothing works/what works paradigm described by Richard Shuker has led to an overwhelming predominance of cognitive behavioural programmes (CBT), which seek to bear down on closely defined aspects of behaviour and thinking and take no note of the whole person or of the impact upon him of his previous life. To many clinicians it is clear that such programmes can have a beneficial but limited effect but it is equally obvious that they are sometimes banal and simplistic and arouse scorn from prisoners, at least when they are out of earshot of their instructors. Recent research is beginning to indicate that earlier highly optimistic treatment effects are not standing the test of time.[5] This is to be expected and is a familiar pattern with 'new revolutionary' treatments, from leeches to Prozac. My hope is that this new realism will allow for the development of true multidisciplinary working within correctional services.

The nature of evidence

At the heart of this conflict is a debate about the nature of evidence and this goes back to the dispute between psychoanalysis and behaviourism. This dispute sometimes seems to be as much about personalities and power structures as the reality of effective treatment. Is cognitive behavioural therapy really a new paradigm? That is to say, is it sufficiently unprecedented to attract an enduring group of adherents away from competing modes of scientific enquiry whilst at the same time leaving plenty of scope for further research?[6] Despite initial appearances, CBT appears to be researching itself back closer to more humanistic approaches, recognising that the client/ therapist relationship is crucial, beginning to understand the implications of transference and adopting concepts such as attachment theory. Agnes Petocz offers a thorough critique of these issues and argues for a breaking down of pseudo-boundaries between different approaches and for a recognition of the equal value of qualitative and quantitative studies.

The structure of the book

The first part of the book looks at some of the central issues that are current in this field. Hans Toch sets the scene and points out some of the essential rules for working with the group he names 'disturbed disruptives'. This interesting term strips the humbug from the more usual euphemisms and enables us to see the importance of labelling in helping us to willingly misunderstand the essence of the individual.

Each of these chapters relates directly to practice but is primarily considering the issue from a theoretical starting point. Mark Morris offers a perspective on the notion of psychopathy which neatly draws out the conceptualisations of different approaches and is able to illustrate how these influence their practice. Practice is central to Richard Shuker's chapter on 'Changing people with programmes'. This was a working title I set him, quite expecting a pained rebuttal and the suggestion of something more impressive such as 'Using a programme approach to rectify the criminogenic features of offenders'. In fact he thought that, plain and straightforward, this is what he wanted to describe and to advocate. As well as providing a most helpful explanation of the theoretical underpinning of the CBT programmes approach, his clinical example would entitle the chapter to appear in Part Two of the book.

The same might be said the other way round with Gillian Proctor's cogent elucidation of the person-centred approach (PCA) to working with dangerous people. Although the theoretical content is high and the chapter contains a powerful critique of social values which circumscribe and mould these behaviours, it seemed important nevertheless that the PCA should reside with other clinical chapters in Part Two.

Three of the chapters in Part Two provide intensely personal testament to the nature of this work. Andrew Downie describes the power of a large group and the nature of the drama which can act as a container for hurt, painful and dangerous feelings. In 'Working with the unbearable', Liz McLure allows us into the intense, private space of the small group. The work she describes is extremely painful, suffused with anger and regret. I know of no other writing which gets so closely to grips with the disturbing dynamics which occur when working with such a disturbed group of men. Finally in this group, Jane Coltman writes about her work as a prison officer. Such a text from a front-line worker is rare and provides a valuable insight into the stresses and rewards of working with this group of men.

The remaining five chapters in Part Two fill in the picture and extend our knowledge that bit further. Jinnie Jeffries is the outstanding psychodramatist in the field of forensic psychotherapy. She has worked at Grendon Prison for many years, has held workshops all over the world and has written numerous papers. Her work, which takes her client group to emotional areas they have avoided for many, many years, takes great courage and her chapter is just a taster of this. Catherine Appleton and Michael Parker provide research-based chapters. Michael Parker examines the relationship between sexual abuse and subsequent offending while Catherine Appleton reports preliminary research findings providing a unique insight into the supervision process of life-sentenced offenders and identifying significant factors that improve the prospect of successful resettlement. Celia Taylor tells of the additional, complicating factors around younger people who appear to pose a risk to themselves or others and highlights the lack of treatment provision.

Finally, Jones and Shuker present a model for the humane treatment of those described as dangerous people. Increasingly we have to justify the work that we do and provide proof that we are doing it correctly. This is no doubt testing for many of us and we may respond testily, but there is some benefit to be gained from this and the UK prison service, through its accreditation process, is in a position to describe in great detail what should happen in their therapeutic communities. This is most important, since therapeutic communities are the treatment setting of choice for this demanding and anxiety provoking group.

It will not have escaped the notice of any reader that many of the contributors to this volume work at, or have worked at, Grendon Prison. Those who do not meet that description have all, or almost all, visited Grendon. The reason is clear. Grendon has been operating as a Therapeutic Community Prison for over 40 years. These have not been easy years. During that time described as the 'nothing works' period Grendon continued to operate. During the chill years of the Thatcher governments, Grendon continued to operate. It is often spoken of as the 'Jewel in the Crown' of the English prison system. It is a model of decency and respect. Yet as that, it inevitably stands as a criticism of practically every other prison in the service. This is an uncomfortable position to be in, for it is bound to arouse envy and resentment from all sides. Nevertheless the question remains: 'why do all other prisons not do as much as Grendon in this respect?'[7]

References

1   Kubik J and Moran J (2003) Lethal elections: gubernatorial politics and the timing of executions. *The Journal of Law & Economics*. **1**: 46.

2   Bright T and Phillips J (2001) Execution of justice. *Birmingham Post Herald*. **December 14–18**.

3   Warren F *et al.* (2003) *Review of treatments for severe personality disorder*. Home Office Online Report, March 30.

4   Cordess C and Cox M (1996) *Forensic Psychotherapy*. Jessica Kingsley, London.

5   Falshaw L, Friendship C, Travers R *et al.* (2003) Searching for 'What Works': an evaluation of cognitive skills programmes. *Findings*. **206**. HM Prison Service Research, Development and Statistics Directorate.

6   Kuhn T (1962) *The Structure of Scientific Revolutions*. The University of Chicago Press, Chicago.

7   Robertson G and Gunn J (1987) A ten year follow up of men discharged from Grendon Prison. *British Journal of Psychiatry*. **151**: 674–8.

Part One

Mainly theory

Chapter 1

The disturbed disruptive

Hans Toch

One of my most frustrating past experiences was an encounter with a group of 'intake analysts' who had been assigned to work at a new reception centre of a large prison system. Among the tools that were to be used by the group was a paper-and-pencil instrument with whose inception I had been associated, which the analysts were to deploy to gauge the degree of compatibility between incoming inmates and the prison settings in which they were to be placed.[1] Determining the initial placement of prisoners is the primary function of intake analysts, so I expected my presentation to be attended with eager anticipation. Instead, the group waited for me to get through my routine so that they could ask a question of obvious interest to them. I forget exactly how they phrased it, but it ran something like: 'What we really want to know is, how can your gizmo help us to differentiate mentally ill inmates from non-mentally ill inmates?' I told them that I couldn't help them do that, but that I felt their pain, since they obviously needed to divest themselves as fast as possible of any clients they could relegate to someone else – in this case, to mental health staff.

The object of the intake exercise at the time was to create a bifurcated process, stratified by the complexity of the inmates' problem. The procedure was one of triage. Some offenders were to be set aside for closer scrutiny by a group of close scrutinisers, while the rest were to be treated to routine classification, and given the proverbial bum's rush. There was no presumption that intake analysts were skilled diagnosticians, but they were presumed to recognise inmates calling for diagnostic acumen. Mostly, what they were expected to do and what they did was rely on diagnoses that had resulted from past encounters with mental health professionals. Recorded stays in a hospital were the most commonly used criterion for referral. If an inmate listed his birthplace as Saturn or Mars he might also qualify – unless the analyst thought he was kidding – and any talk of suicide was a statutorily mandated cue.

The skilled diagnosticians largely ratified the judgement of the unskilled diagnosticians, except that they were less impressed with talk of suicide because they were experienced (and therefore cynical) professionals. But once the inmates had been twice – and now, officially – labelled, they were ready to be placed in close proximity to mental health services, which meant that they were assigned to maximum security prisons, where such services were located. At this point the inmates had arrived in their prison of residence with credentials that certified their prospective entitlement to a diagnosis of mental illness, should the occasion arise.

Underselling pathology

For the inmates in question, the best sort of occasion for them to mobilise their status as mentally ill prisoners was to manifest symptoms that did not violate any institutional rules, though this is admittedly difficult to accomplish. Quiet hallucinations or outlandish delusions would of course serve nicely, provided they were not obtrusive but became ultimately noticeable. A nice, textbook depression would be ideal, but a suicide attempt could be risky, on at least three counts: First, it was apt to constitute a disciplinary violation; and second, crusty clinicians often regarded self-injuries as flagrant manipulative behaviour. Lastly, there was always a chance of unforeseen lethality.

One reason why prisoners were ill-advised to manifest symptoms that violated institutional rules (ranging from inconveniently sloppy housekeeping to serious tantrums) was that this would create taxonomic confusion, and could place the inmates' status as mental patients in jeopardy. The prisoners could be particularly at risk of muddying the waters if they had committed destructive acts in the past and been convicted of violent offences. Violent offenders who become disruptive in prison invite particular attention to the damage they can do rather than to their motivation for doing it. This perspective understandably extends to apprehensive clinicians to whom the disruptive inmates are referred, who can deploy special labels (such as 'character disorder' or 'psychopathic personality') to communicate the fact that they are personally concerned about the harm a person has been perpetrating, and consequently indifferent to the admittedly consistent eccentricity of his behaviour. More or less pejorative clinical labels qualify as diagnostic categories, but do not invite the delivery of mental health assistance.[2] Instead, they communicate the opposite message, which is something like, 'Don't bring this person to me, because he is obviously more bad than mad, and therefore not within my purview.'

Badness pre-empts, especially in prisons. One reason for this pre-emption is that offenders are assumed to earn their way into prison by being bad persons, just as others earn their way into hospitals by being sick. This preconception is plausible, but it makes no provision for individuals who are sent to prison because they have engaged in disturbed behaviour that violates the law, or for the many offenders who are clearly emotionally or intellectually handicapped.[3] It is also obvious that in prisons disruptive behaviour gets priority attention because the goals of maintaining order and preserving security have become self-contained ends. In many prisons, rule enforcing is an obsessive preoccupation of uniformed and civilian staff. Almost invariably, the verbalised justifications for punishing prison-rule violators consist of mantras, such as 'you have endangered the order and safety of the facility'. Such formulations leave little room for extended ruminations about the perpetrator's hypothetical motives.

Disruptiveness also happens to be the most salient attribute of much symptomatic behaviour. In any setting in which people live in close proximity to each other, one man's unscheduled conduct is liable to disrupt another's routine, which is not a recipe for garnering popularity. And symptoms of mental illness are not only reliably spontaneous, but tend to be loud, messy, assertive, irritating and unresponsive to conciliatory overtures. In settings that are redolent with rules, it also becomes impossible to display symptoms of mental illness without violating dozens of proscriptions and prohibitions. Moreover, regimes that are inhospitable to eccentricity bring out the worst in many patients. Disruptive behaviour earns punishment, and punishment is apt to make sick people sicker. Disturbed-disruptive offenders frequently become more disturbed when they are dealt with as disruptive offenders, and are liable to become more disruptive when they become more disturbed. This means that punishing disturbed-disruptive offenders can be an open invitation to distressing boomerang effects.

Punishment as iatrogenic treatment

As a rule, the social isolation and enforced inactivity of segregation settings present insurmountable stressors to even moderately disturbed prisoners,[4] though there are some very disturbed persons who may find conditions of stimulus-reduction ameliorative. These mentally ill persons can therefore survive in segregation settings, if vegetating meets one's criterion of survival. At the other extreme, however, many degenerative escalations can be observed. Punishment in prisons mostly means extended segregated confinement, which invites reactions such out-of-control panic or rage. When such feelings are translated into behaviour, they can lead to additional punishment and consequently to further disruptive behaviour. At the culmination of such a cycle, the prisoner may have become a redoubtable monster, and his keepers may wallow in impotence and in understandable despair. Every prison system has prisoners deemed unmanageable by acclamation, and most qualify as disturbed as well as disruptive.

The fact that prison staff members react punitively to disruptiveness, and tend to undersell the mental health problems of disruptive (and, especially, violent) inmates, may be lamentable, but it does not imply that these prisoners would be better off if they were dealt with as disturbed and limited attention were paid to their disruptive behaviour. For one, such a view would be wildly distorted. Typically, disturbed-disruptive offenders are multi-problem offenders, who have lived chequered lives featuring multifarious and unimpressive delinquency, chronic homelessness and variegated substance abuse.[5] Beyond repeated mental health contacts that have frequently been initiated at early ages, such individuals tend to have other institutional experiences reliably marked by failure – usually at least partly due to the manifestation of chronically disruptive behaviour. The behaviour may vary in kind, but its psychological impact ranges from being blatantly dysfunctional to being self-destructive as well as destructive to others.

Prescriptive implications

Any prospect of ameliorating the unimpressive lot of disturbed-disruptive offenders hinges on the ability to modify the contribution the offender makes to his own downhill career. This means that we must remain focused on the offender's destructive involvements. In retaining this focus, we must make a point of acting on the behaviour, rather than reacting to it, as customarily occurs. The disruptive offender is habituated to the aversive responses that he reliably engenders. Rejections have become grist for his mill, undergirding his hostility, feeding his contrariness and cementing his practised posture of sullen resentfulness. The first order of business, therefore, must be to break through the offender's stance.[6] This means that we must undermine his unconscious preconceptions, which feed his view of himself as a perennial victim of a perversely inhospitable world.

This task of disconfirmation is a difficult one if we attempt it in a conventional prison. Even if we act consistently non-punitive and non-rejecting, others can be relied upon to subvert our campaign. To succeed, we have to control enough of the offender's environment to prevent enactment of the rejecting-parent role, which is almost second nature to prison staff members. The offender exposed to our message should have to experience the shock and surprise of not being able to engender any of the aversive responses he expects. He should have to become sufficiently unsettled to become receptive to therapeutic intervention (irrespective of modality), a state that in clinical parlance is traditionally called a 'transference'.[7]

To work with any disturbed-disruptive offender, we have to try to understand his pattern of disruptive behaviour, because we need to understand this pattern if we are to help the offender to understand himself. Uncontaminated understanding requires that one not be blinded by preconceptions implicit in scintillating diagnostic labels to which we may be deeply attached. It also requires that we not become preoccupied by the distractingly horrendous violence the offender may have perpetrated. We must keep in mind that each offender's pattern of conduct is fundamentally unique, reflecting his own set of inappropriate feelings and skewed perceptions and clumsy or destructive approaches to interpersonal dilemmas. Such perspectives can be explored through immersions in accounts of the offender's misbehaviour.

We must concurrently familiarise ourselves with situations in which the person has acted disruptively, to understand the antecedents of his violence. The goal of such preparatory inquiry is not to end up sharing our insights with the offender, which would be an impressive but predictably pointless endeavour. We need pattern-related information as a source of hypotheses to be tested as we go along working with the offender, for case conferences concerned with the offender, as a way of anticipating situations that we are likely to encounter as we challenge the offender's coping capacity, and to gauge the offender's eventual progress in therapy. We also need pattern-related information to resolve issues related to group dynamics, starting with the composition of groups.

Groups are advantageous in dealing with disturbed-disruptive offenders, for any number of reasons. For one, it is easier – and more inviting – to note dysfunctional behaviour in others before one sees it in oneself. And in self-exploration, a group can serve as validator, as audience and a source of consensus, testifying to insights and buttressing resolves. An important advantage of groups is that they can enforce structure and discipline with impunity, without the baggage of the inevitable negative transference evoked by direct top-down exercises of authority. Whether we like it or not, behavioural rules must be spelled out in detail, and must be consistently enforced. This is a requisite for any intervention with offenders, but must become a key feature when we work with offenders whose institutional rule-breaking is a target of treatment. If we want to explore and address rule-breaking, there must be rules to be broken, and violations of rules that occur must be taken seriously. We may prefer a permissive environment, but in such a milieu we would have little to discuss with the offender, who would be unable to engage in misbehaviour serendipitously reminiscent of past transgressions and revelatory of behavioural patterning.

Therapy groups invite the enactment of the golden rule because as a group member I can do unto you what you have done unto me, which ought to deter bullying and scapegoating. However, the process is not automatic, and must be reinforced by skilled leadership. Skilled leadership is also required to discourage the innumerable forms of conscious and unconscious filibuster that groups use to make sure that nothing gets done.[8] And most importantly, group discussion must be guided – firmly but gently – so that at the end of the day analytic discourse yields plausible inferences about the dynamics of behaviour.

Disturbed-disruptive offenders require multidisciplinary treatment, and programmes for such offenders are best run by an interdisciplinary staff, working as teams. Teaming at its best involves the abrogation of role definitions, with each team member contributing what he can as an individual, regardless of disciplinary affiliation. Clinical expertise obviously matters when one works with disturbed-disruptive offenders, but knowledge can be shared with others in the course of joint endeavours. Such sharing of knowledge is sometimes called 'training', but terms are not important. Maxwell Jones, the progenitor of the therapeutic community, was fond of saying that he had treated his staff and trained his patients. Where our goal is to promote change, the process we engender is learning, and this process at its best must involve all the members of any treatment community.

References

1   Toch H (1992) *Living in Prison: the ecology of survival.* American Psychological Association (APA Books), Washington, DC.

2   Toch H (1998) Psychopathy or antisocial personality in forensic settings. In: T Millon, E Simonson, M Birket-Smith and R Davis (eds) *Psychopathy: antisocial, criminal and violent behavior.* The Guilford Press, New York and London.

3   Toch H and Adams K (2002) *Acting Out: maladaptive behavior in confinement.* American Psychological Association (APA Books), Washington, DC.

4   Haney C (2003) Mental health issues in long-term solitary and 'supermax' confinement. *Crime and Delinquency.* **49**(1): 124–56.

5   Toch H and Adams K (1994) *The Disturbed Violent Offender.* American Psychological Association (APA Books), Washington, DC.

6   Cullen E (1997) Can a prison be a therapeutic community? The Grendon template. In: E Cullen, L Jones and R Woodward (eds) *Therapeutic Communities for Offenders.* Wiley, Chichester.

7   Aichhorn A (1955) *Wayward Youth.* Meridian Books, New York.

8   Bion WR (1961) *Experience in Groups and Other Papers.* Tavistock, London.

Chapter 2

Some ethical issues in psychodynamic work with dangerous people

Mark Morris

There is an idea that the moral valence of a society can be determined by the way it treats its criminals. Although this is something of a sound bite for the penal reformists, this test of the general level of collective decency is actually quite sophisticated. By and large, the criminal population themselves will have acted in a morally reprehensible way, at least in relation to the index offence for which they are detained. They will be guilty of riding roughshod over the rights of their fellow man, and in so doing might be argued to have surrendered any claim to ethical treatment by the society that they have offended. The concept of morality seems never far from the surface in the management of dangerous people by criminal justice agencies. For example, the moral questions raised by accounts of offending have led to an understanding of psychopathy that proposes the syndrome to be a disorder of moral development. While this may be supported by a contemporary psychological meta-theory, of course the notion of criminals as in some way morally bankrupt or degenerate is traditional. The UK Prison Act that requires a vicar to be retained for a prison to operate articulates this perspective, as do the variety of missions to the 'fallen'.

Interesting though the relation between moral development and criminality is, it is not the subject of this chapter. The focus here is more on the ethical issues surrounding the treatment of difficult and dangerous people, not about whether it is legitimate to act morally towards those who have acted immorally to others. That one should act morally with this group is taken as a given. The subject of this chapter is to explore the morality of aspects of trying to treat such people.

Incarceration

There is an old school style of prison governor, who, while proud of their life's work in prisons, is all too aware of the trauma and deprivation that a prison term inflicts on people. Wistfully, they look forward to a day when no longer do one group of people need to lock up another group. 'There must be a better way.' Ironically, over the last two decades, there has indeed been a growth in an alternative not requiring long-term imprisonment, namely execution. It is a sobering thought that probably the bulk of patients I have worked closely and struggled with in prison settings would have been executed in some jurisdictions. From this perspective, paradoxically, long-term incarceration can be seen as an articulation of a society's decency.

Broadly, the ethical justifications for the incarceration of criminals are threefold. First is that the deprivation of liberty is a punishment for whatever the crime or misdemeanour has been. The punishment is retribution for the wrong. In this model, the length of the sentence is specifically determined by the severity of the crime. There are two problems with this approach in practice, the main one being that an attitude of punishment is difficult to maintain in reality. The reality of custodial environments is that there are a large number of potentially violent people locked up in close proximity, and outnumbering and with less to lose than the custodians. To manage such settings, the covert consent of the criminal client group is imperative. To achieve this, custody is framed in terms of rehabilitation, prisoners' rights and so on. In spite of this difficulty of maintaining a retributive punishment focus in the real world, as an ethical proposition, namely that incarceration is a punishment, one to 'fit' the crime and cancel it out somehow – 'paying the debt to society' – this is a particularly persuasive argument, impervious to the criticism that 'two wrongs don't make a right'.

The second main ethical justification can be developed from a utilitarian perspective. In short, this would acknowledge that the deprivations inflicted by incarceration are indeed an evil – so defined because they cause suffering. The utilitarian justification would be that the evil and suffering caused by incarceration is outweighed by the suffering caused by allowing the dangerous person freedom to carry on their violent lifestyle.

This account of the ethical justification of incarceration makes the case in terms of the suffering prevented of future potential victims. A further justification can be made in terms of potential benefits to the incarcerated individual themselves if criminal behaviour is conceived of as an illness. While this idea might initially seem outlandish, it does have some merit. Traditionally, the whole basis of the criminal justice process rests on the notion of criminal choice – mens rea – a mind that made a decision to execute an illegal act. However, the concept of personality disorder – where an individual's attitudes and behaviours are themselves the pathology – and antisocial personality or psychopathic personality in particular – where the characteristic pathology consists of violent and irresponsible conduct – can begin to reframe the issue of criminal behaviour into a medical problem.

The ethical justification of incarceration on the basis of personality disorder goes something like this. For the psychopathic individual, offences or adverse incidents are the manifest pathology, and constitute harm to the individual. In a controlled prison environment, the opportunities and freedom of the individual are curtailed, and the probability of their committing such crimes is reduced. Control of psychopathic behaviour in a custodial environment thus prevents a deterioration of the psychopathic condition, and can be conceived as a form of treatment, beneficial to the individual.

Bleak, monotonous, boring and depriving as prison environments can be, there is at least an argument that they provide a regular and balanced diet, access to medical and dental care, relative protection from the excesses of drug use, and relative protection from the excesses of gangland culture and violence. Concretely, for many chaotic people whose lifestyle revolves around drug use, survival rates in prison may exceed those in the community, where access to drugs, violence and chaos is much greater.

The restriction of an individual's psychopathic behaviour can be conceived of as a psychological therapeutic intervention – a behavioural therapy if you will. Within secure settings, there are available a number of other treatment options and approaches. Broadly, these have been characterised as follows. Beyond the behavioural intervention of the prevention of psychopathic behaviour by the prison wall on one hand, there is the 'adjudication system' for trying and punishing bad behaviour, and the 'token economy' of the incentives and earned privileges scheme, where acceptable behaviour is rewarded with additions to what people are allowed; for example, a television in the cell. Both of these promote and encourage good behaviour. Moving on into the cognitive realm, the 'What Works' movement has spawned a raft of psychological programmes that combine a cognitive ideology with a didactic style of delivery to groups of prisoners, looking at specific tasks such as cognitive skills, and sex offending. There is no doubt that these programmes are effective and helpful, although their delivery can be criticised as being formulaic, and the process of 'meeting offending behaviour needs' using them has become concretised.

Third, there are a series of more psychodynamic programmes, less so the drug therapeutic communities that derive from a 12-step self-help ideology, but more so the Grendon and Dovegate therapeutic communities in the UK, described in some of the chapters in this volume. These settings have as a central vision the application of group therapeutic principles in a residential setting leading to a 'democratic' therapeutic community ethos. It is with issues relating to such treatment that this volume is concerned, and with the ethical issues thrown up by such treatment settings that the bulk of this chapter is concerned.

Consent

In medical school teaching regarding the ethical dimension to practice, the question is posed about what the difference is between a surgeon's knife cutting the skin, and a criminal assailant with a switchblade in a dark alley. The answer is consent. The patient consents to the surgeon cutting them, but does not consent to the assailant. The fact is that most medical and more broadly therapeutic interventions are assault until and unless consent for the procedure is granted.

Subsequent case law has established that not only is consent necessary, but also this consent needs to be adequately informed. If a patient signs up to an operation under the illusion that there will be no complications, without an adequate knowledge of the potential risks involved, this is not true consent. Informed consent is required prior to laying a hand on a patient to do anything.

In setting out the context for a discussion on consent in the treatment of violent people, there is a third piece of the jigsaw. The old adage that 'sticks and stones will break my bones, but words will never hurt me' is emphatically dead. There is now a clear equivalence between physical violence (sticks and stones) and psychological violence (words). In some cases, society reviles psychological violence more than physical. Much of the moral panic about sex offending is related to this. In handing down a prison sentence to a man who gropes a woman's breasts on a London bus, the main damage that is done is not physical, it is mental: the psychological trauma of an overt sexual act taking place without her consent; the destruction of the woman's sense of personal security to ride the buses, secure that she will not be molested; the destruction of the woman's sense of control and integrity over her own physical body, amplified by the particularity of sexual privacy. This equivalence of psychological and physical violence is also seen in the civil courts, with litigation payouts for instances of bullying, harassment and psychological trauma. This has relevance to the application of the psychological therapies. It establishes that a psychological therapy is potentially an assault if the patient does not consent to be treated.

There is no doubt that the truth can be traumatic. Peoples' lives are built on the foundations of what they believe about themselves, not necessarily what is true about themselves. The trauma of learning that a spouse has been unfaithful; the trauma of learning that one has been adopted; these examples represent truths that undermine an individual's believed reality. As the belief is challenged and shown to be false, there is a psychological crisis leading to a self re-evaluation.

The potency of psychodynamic psychotherapy as a treatment method rests on its ability to define an individual's belief systems about themselves, to understand this by reference to their history and experiences, then to challenge the false beliefs. This process, while beneficial in the longer term by enabling people to more rationally manage themselves, in the short term can be extremely disturbing and disabling. In some cases, the process can be damaging, for example with some psychotic patients.

Psychodynamic psychotherapy deconstructs fixed incorrect belief systems that are impeding the individual. If, for example, an individual is hostile and suspicious to all men with beards, and their boss has a beard, then a psychodynamic treatment might explore why this might be so – emerging with a hypothesis that a rather dodgy teacher at primary school and one of father's dodgy friends both had beards, so that a belief has developed that dodgy men to be suspicious of have beards.

The deconstructing of this belief will have three effects. First, it will re-awaken the trauma of the experience with the dodgy characters in the past. This will be more or less traumatic depending on the nature of the memory. For example, if school was a wretched experience with endemic bullying and frank abuse from the dodgy teacher, a memory that has been able to be forgotten by virtue of avoiding bearded men, the recall of this possible reason for the false belief might itself be quite traumatic.

Second, it will increase a general sense of insecurity. The nice thing about the false belief that all dodgy characters have beards is that they can be easily spotted and avoided. If dodginess and facial hair are in fact independent characteristics, then how can one keep safe from them? This issue crystallises the defensive function of the false belief. The belief protects the individual from something, some threat or fear, in this case from the potential harm from certain people. It may be that in further working through it becomes clear, for example, that the fear is overestimated, and that there are not as many dodgy characters in the world as the individual believes, they were just unlucky as a child, or some other understanding. Either way, the point still remains that a defensive, protective belief will have been collapsed, and that this may itself be experienced as a trauma in the short term, and will be generally destabilising.

From a psychodynamic perspective, one of the understandings of psychosis is that the mind is overly porous; that the delusional beliefs and hallucinatory experiences of the psychotic are the daydreams and internal conversations of the non-psychotic. Psychosis demonstrates a difficulty in differentiating reality from fantasy. Defensive structures such as the example above, while not entirely accurate, do provide a grasp on reality, a handhold that allows life to be engaged with. For some, psychological defences are not an irritant that gets in the way of a better life, they are the underpinning that prevents them falling away into a psychotic abyss. There is always a risk that deconstructing some of these defensive false beliefs will make a precarious psychological situation worse. For example, if dodgy people do not have beards, and anyone may be dodgy, this could lead to rather a paranoid reaction of widespread suspicion and fear.

The third, and hoped for, effect of deconstructing the belief about men with beards might be that the individual can function more effectively with their bearded boss, be less vulnerable to beard-free dodgy characters, and be more aware of the workings of their own psychology and the effects of their historical experiences. Should this occur, it will have been at a considerable cost to the individual, namely the process of trauma of insight and recollection; and it will be via a process that is not without risk of psychological harm. Consequently, there is a need in such psychological therapies to be clear about establishing consent.

In clinical practice with more severely personality-disordered characters this dynamic seems to take a particular form. For example, a borderline patient who regularly self-harms and cuts will start a treatment programme with a set of symptoms that is harrowing to friends, family and professional workers. But the individual themselves may have no particular complaints, and may be contemptuous and critical of all the fuss that is being made. If successful, treatment will enable them to see why they cut, what feelings they manage by terrorising people in their surroundings, and for the individual, this might be quite difficult to bear. As the meaning and the defensive role of the symptom is explored, for example via confrontation of the terror that the self-cutter can inflict on those close to them, the underlying issues will emerge, and can begin to be explored. Gradually, the self-cutting will recede as the individual faces the real underlying issues – often very complex and difficult; often more difficult than the relative simplicity of cutting safely. As one patient put it at the end of treatment, '. . . when I came here I was fine, I just carved up. Now I'm miserable.'

With people whose symptoms are more to do with violence – for example those serving long prison sentences for violent offences – the picture is similar. The majority of violent offenders do not see their violence as a problem, they see it as a solution; they see it as their strength and their main asset. They are contemptuous of those 'pussies' who do not share a stereotypical macho view of the world. The gender role reference is informative and, although derogatory, is worth articulating. A 'pussy' in prison parlance is a man who is soft and yielding, even caring and feminine, someone who can be overcome, or who does not stand up. There is a link between the slang term for female genitalia 'pussy' and these characteristics of particular men. As a psychiatrist or psychotherapist in a prison setting, I am a 'pussy' for these reasons, because I do not actively avow the stereotypical macho culture where violence is idealised.

In the course of treatment, the violent person in treatment first has to recognise a difference between potency and violence. There is an enormous narcissistic wound when the violent person finally recognises that in spite of being a 'pussy' I can say things that have relevance, validity and genuinely perceived potency, that I can be potent as a 'pussy' rather than as part of the rubbished coercive force of the 'strong arm of the law', which is always perceived as only having got the upper hand 'this time'. The second trauma is becoming aware that beneath the big, frightening, violent, bullying exterior, they too are 'pussies'. They too have vulnerabilities, sensitivities, unhappiness, regrets and all those things that have been disavowed for so long. For violent people, in some ways the macho, violent solution is certainly simpler, and in the short term easier, than having to face the reality of personal fallibility, vulnerability and insecurity. They too can feel that they were 'fine' until they engaged in treatment. Before, all their problems were sorted out in the showers (a favoured site for prison fights). After, things are much more difficult.

Informed consent: insight and risk

Informed consent is something of a holy grail; how can one have a full understanding of the medical or surgical treatment options for a condition without being a doctor or a surgeon, and an expert versed in the latest literature at that? Even by qualifying the expectation with the rider that the consentee is 'reasonably informed', the requirement in practice has been somewhat cynically reduced to a medico-legal, self-defensive sound bite, with the patient given the percentage survival or cure rates for the different treatments, and invited to make a choice.

Within the psychodynamic therapies, however, the problem is compounded by two further issues; the lack of empirical evidence of efficacy, and the problems with informing the patient about the nature of treatment.

The problems surrounding the use of empirical data to inform patients are present in more medical psychiatry also. At a best guess, for a moderately depressed person, treatment with antidepressants will improve the mood of a third, make no difference for a third, and make a third worse. For psychological treatments, there is more evidence of the efficacy of short-term cognitive treatments in relation to their identified treatment target, but much less evidence about longer term effects, or broader improvement outwith the narrow band of the psychological symptom. With the psychodynamic treatments, the situation is even worse, in part because of the variety of effects described above. Is it reasonable to describe the substitution of a self-cutting symptom for a more subdued depressive picture as an improvement? Arguably, the cognitive therapies are effective by shoring up defences, by strengthening rationalisations – for example, there is no rational reason to be afraid of spiders in the UK.

Arguably, the psychodynamic therapies are of a nature that the treatment effect cannot be adequately investigated by empirical methodologies. The process is too individual, too focused on the individual client, their developmental history and particular personal psychopathology to be generalisable.

Part of the problem with looking at outcome in the psychodynamic therapies is in defining what would be a good outcome in the first place, and this relates to the second issue pertaining to the difficulties in informing consent. If you ask a person post psychodynamic therapy what treatment is like, they are likely to stare into the middle distance and be lost for words, or at best say that they don't know how to describe it, or even that they can be sure if it did 'work', although they will usually acknowledge that things are different somehow.

Psychodynamic therapy is principally a relationship employed for therapeutic benefit. Like personal relationships, it is something that simply *is*, something that is difficult to describe. Some of the effects of this relationship can be identified. Gradually the parties in the relationship get to know and understand each other. For the patient, they are helped to understand aspects of their own experience and psychopathology by sharing in the understanding that the therapist has. In turn, their therapist's understanding is derived from their (the therapist's) understanding of their own, similar psychopathology. In addition, the therapist begins to understand the patient better, and to learn about them, both in terms of historical facts, and in terms of the way that they function more broadly.

For offender and violent populations, knowledge of history and an understanding of psychological functioning are central aspects of risk assessment. So a psychodynamic treatment might potentially throw up rich material related to risk assessment. The issue of confidentiality will be discussed below, but the current point is that in consenting to treatment, the individual needs to be aware that previously hidden aspects are likely to emerge.

This issue – an emergence of a greater self-knowledge and awareness – is not unproblematic. In the current risk assessment cultural environment, it seems that the more that is known about people, the higher their level of risk is assumed to be. In the adversarial judicial process, the task of the individual's barrister is to establish that there is a reasonable doubt that their client committed the crimes for which they are charged. In part this is achieved by minimising and rationalising the incident. For example, a man charged with murder for a pub brawl where the victim was stabbed and bled to death would develop for the court an account of how this was not his nature, about how this was a playful fight in high spirits that all members of the jury will have been involved in at some time, but an everyday fisticuffs that had gone disastrously wrong.

Say, for example, that the individual receives a conviction for manslaughter rather than murder, because doubt is cast on the mens rea, the intent, and that they then come into a psychodynamic therapeutic process in which the account of the offending and its contextual mindset are considerably expanded. Perhaps the truth emerges that the individual has been obsessed with killing, has had fantasies for years about what it might be like to kill, and has spent years planning and trying to engineer fights and risky situations. Say that the long-standing fantasy has been to find a bullying and boorish bigger man, start a fight, then bring out a knife, and delight in the momentary recognition in the big man's face of surprise and fear in the seconds before the knife is plunged in. Such an account would escalate the individual's perceived risk factors to sky high, possibly putting back many years their opportunity for release on parole or licence.

This would be an example where the therapeutic process of exploration and expansion brings out a truth that may not be in the patient's interests. An honest truth emerges about an individual that casts them in a much worse light that had been anticipated. As a result of the therapeutic exploration, the individual is materially worse off after treatment than they were before.

Allied to this problem of potentially adverse disclosure is the problem of unconvicted offences. There is a truism with the phenomenon of breaking the law, that the actual offence only represents the tip of the iceberg; that usually, to get caught for something, you must have been doing it lots of times and not getting caught. To be able to engage in a realistic discourse about oneself, there is a need to be open about such activity. It is difficult to understand a life pattern without gaining an impression of some historical data; it is difficult to understand how a bank robber moved from house burglaries to post offices and on to banks if there is nothing on the criminal record pertaining to houses or post offices, and there is no possibility of disclosure of the historical marker points along the way.

Practically, there is a partial solution to the specific problem of the need to talk about unconvicted crimes, namely the 'TPP' rule. 'TPP' refers to the specific information about the time, the place and the persons involved in a crime. Experience suggests that the police are not particularly interested in chasing around trying to guess the details of long past, unsolved crimes without some fairly specific information, which would include the time and date, the place and the people involved. So unconvicted offences can be discussed without specific details emerging, which allows staff to engage in the accounts without having to immediately report to the police all the intelligence that they are receiving.

If one solution to the therapeutic dilemma of the need to talk about unconvicted crime in the attempt to get closer to the truth in the psycho-dynamic treatment of such dangerous people is to be a bit fuzzy about the specifics, the other solution is to come clean. To own up – to take the rap, to get it off one's chest and face the music.

Embracing the truth in the form of owning up to previous offending provides a model for the way out of the ethical dilemma posed above. In the example above, the pub killer's perceived risk status was ratcheted up by the disclosure of a sadistic and macabre fantasy context to the offence. It may actually be the case that the risk has been reduced.

Such fantasies are usually buried deep inside the individual, because of an awareness of their grotesqueness and perversity. The fact that such a fantasy system has been exposed, has been brought into the light of day – encountered by a person other than the victim – in itself considerably reduces the risk of it being enacted. First, by being shared, it has a discursive realm in which to be manifest extra-psychically. Until such a disclosure, the only opportunity for outward manifestation was actual enactment. The push to enact can henceforth be forestalled by talking.

Second, it is characteristic that such fantasies are two-person – the perpetrator and victim/s. Disclosure considerably reduces the power and intensity of the fantasy by introducing a third person – the observer or therapist to whom the disclosure has been made. In part, this reduction in risk derives from the developmental difference between a pre-Oedipal, primitive object relating, and a more mature post-Oedipal situation. Part of the toxicity of the fantasy is removed by virtue of disclosure moving it on a developmental stage.

The third problem with the approach to risk assessment where evidence of offensive fantasy increases concern is that, from a psychoanalytic perspective, we all have pretty offensive fantasy lives. Psychoanalytically, dreams and daydreams represent wishes. A man who dreams about the death of his wife is expressing a murderous fantasy about her even though he may disown and be traumatised by the dream; our enjoyment of action films with a high body count articulates our own murderous violence. Our collective disapprobation for sex offenders, while following lurid real life accounts of sex crimes, articulates our own disavowed perverse wishes.

If a psychoanalytic account of human nature is true, then perverse and violent fantasy is ubiquitous, and finding it in an offender is unremarkable. Indeed, the opposite may be true – not finding such fantasy material would shed doubt on the validity of the individual's account.

While these criticisms of fantasy-based risk assessment have some legitimacy within psychodynamic psychotherapy circles, they have little recognition outside. The sad reality is that if an offender in treatment explains what was going through their mind at the time of the offence, and how this relates to other characteristic thoughts and fantasies, they might find themselves viewed as more rather than less of a risk. Volunteers from the offender population need to be aware of these issues as they consent to treatment.

The other way out of this dilemma of disclosure is the development of a general degree of psychological mindedness and insight so that the fantasy itself can be put in context. For example, the man who kills someone in a fight and then discloses a rather more murky set of fantasies about murder might discover a memory of a violent and abusive father. The obsession with killing might have its origin in a repeated threat from the father, while beating him, that he was going to 'kill him this time'. The wish to find a big bully might have a similar paternal explanation.

Often, in such accounts of extreme abuse, as the boy grows into a young adult, a moment occurs where the youth can fight back and win. Physically, the tables are turned, and the father realises that the son has become a physical match. No longer will father be able to take out his frustrations on his son. This moment is one of considerable triumph for the youth, and probably serves to consolidate the belief in violence as an asset. Perhaps this is genesis of the moment of realisation for the knifed bully in the fantasy.

The way out of the ethical disclosure dilemma is to hope that not only can the individual make sufficient progress to articulate the underlying fantasy context of the offence, but also to be able to put the fantasy itself into a context. The fantasy will have a personal and historical meaning that the individual recognises, and can move on from.

Conclusions

In this chapter, a number of the ethical issues that emerge when trying to treat difficult and dangerous people in an exploratory or psychodynamic treatment modality such as Grendon Prison in the UK have been explored. From the perspective of psychoanalytic theory, every person's heart has some pretty dark places. This awareness and knowledge can be used to help more dangerous people understand themselves better, understand some of the things that they have done better, and be able to make choices to try to avoid doing them again.

This process of understanding is not without risk. In some cases, the insight and facing of the dark part of the soul is too much, and cannot be borne; in some cases the illusion is more comforting than the reality, and real life is more difficult than life with the illusion. In some cases, the excavation of truth and insight can in fact work against the individual, making them appear more dangerous. All these are risks of treatment. The benefits of being more self-aware, of understanding better one's history, of putting aside illusions and engaging more with reality – all of these advantages of successful treatment need to be set against the potential problems.

The difficulty is that this summary may have very much more meaning for those who have traversed an exploratory therapeutic process than for those who have not. To be able to fully grasp the ethical dilemmas involved in exploratory psychotherapeutic treatment or to be able to give informed consent, one may need to have engaged with it already.

Chapter 3

Science, meaning and the scientist-practitioner model of treatment

Agnes Petocz

Introduction

In a recent letter to the editor of *The Chronicle of Higher Education*, in response to an article which describes scientists and practising psychologists as engaged in continuing warfare across a 'scientist–therapist gap', Robert Sternberg, the President of the American Psychological Association, accuses the author of misrepresenting almost every aspect of the relationship between practising psychologists and scientists. After pointing out that many psychologists properly view themselves as scientist-practitioners or practitioner-scientists, he adds:

> 'It is simply not the case that scientists make one set of claims, and practitioners another. One of the beauties of science is that it is self-correcting. Science informs practice, but practice also informs science. There is no war between scientists and practitioners. The number of scientifically trained clinicians is growing, not shrinking. Accreditation standards require that psychological practice be based on the science of psychology and that trainees have training in empirically supported procedures regardless of training model. Competent practising psychologists keep up on the science of psychology just as competent practising medical doctors or practising lawyers keep up with their fields. The idea that practitioners generally do not want to be aware of scientific developments is false. Artificially pitting one group against another – in this case, scientists against practitioners – cannot possibly help psychologists or anyone else attain a common good. Today's world has more than its share of useless, senseless wars. There is no need to manufacture or otherwise foment another one.'[1]

Concern with the relationship between science and practice in psychology is not new, and the tensions of the past cannot be denied. However, as Sternberg suggests, the model of the 'scientist-practitioner' has become increasingly prominent. And in this model it is not a case of the scientist being pitted against the practitioner; rather, the division is between the *scientific* practitioner, whose 'evidence-based practice' dutifully adheres to 'empirically supported procedures', and the *other* kind of practitioner – *anti*-scientific, *un*scientific, *pseudo*-scientific, or *not-quite*-scientific.

Let me say at the outset that I agree with the spirit of Sternberg's observations – that promotion of the scientist-practitioner model is justified, and that it should continue to be upheld as the standard for all forms of psychological intervention. However, the implementation of the model is only as good as the conception of science upon which it is based. And, as I shall argue in this chapter, that conception is seriously defective.

In brief, the assumptions underlying the present model are a legacy of psychology's efforts to extricate itself from its philosophical background and attain scientific respectability. In this struggle, mainstream psychology has tended to embrace a number of core beliefs and practices which it takes to be the hallmarks of science, and simultaneously to neglect or marginalise anything which is regarded as incompatible with them. Central among these excluded elements is the concept of *meaning*. As Eysenck put it, 'an approach which stresses *meaning* is the exact opposite of the natural science approach which stresses the study of *behavior*' (p. 194).[2] The resulting tensions – ranging from uneasy alliance to radical schism – between 'science' on the one hand and 'meaning' on the other are reflected in practice in the clashes between putatively scientific and evidence-based treatments, usually behavioural or cognitive behavioural, and enshrined in the scientist-practitioner model, and the more humanistic and psychodynamically-oriented approaches, which employ interpretative techniques to address the 'subjective meanings' and 'lived experiences' held to be central in the psychotherapeutic or psychoanalytic encounter.

My contention is that *scientism* in mainstream psychology has led to widespread and deep misconceptions about two things: the meaning of science, and the science of meaning.[3] As Sternberg is at pains to remind us, practising accredited psychologists are typically trained in academic institutions, as scientists first and as practitioners second, and in accordance with those institutions' prevailing conceptions of science and of scientific evidence. Inevitably, then, misconceptions carry over into the scientist-practitioner model and its application. Those same misconceptions have also handicapped advocates of multidisciplinarity and multifocal treatment approaches; for only with a full appreciation of the meaning of science, and only with a clear understanding of the meaning of meaning and its scientific investigation, can the case for flexibility be vindicated, not (as is typically attempted) by appeals to post-Kuhnian relativism and paradigm incommensurability, but by pointing out just how much, and why, true science would actually *demand* such flexibility.

Furthermore, scientism in psychology has led to the polarisation of attitudes towards science into deification on one side and demonisation on the other. Replacing scientism by genuine science would not only alter the nature and perceptions of the scientist-practitioner model of treatment. It would thereby underscore the place of the model within a coherent integration of recent trends in psychology, particularly the reinvigoration of qualitative research methods, and the emergence of a number of so-called 'revolutions' (consciousness, affective, renewed cognitive, etc). This would provide a necessary buffer against the misunderstandings and distortions which threaten to contaminate even these promising new trends.

Scientistic misconceptions of science and of meaning

Wittgenstein attributed the 'barrenness' of psychology to its mixture of 'experimental methods and *conceptual confusion*' (p. 232).[4] Critics have continued to impugn conceptions *and* methods, charging psychologists with errors born from ignorance of the history, philosophy and logic of science. Some of these errors are: the conflation of empirical realism with positivism;[5-8] obsession with 'operationalisation' and over-zealous adherence to the principle of Ockham's razor, leading to ecological invalidity in many experimental 'findings';[9] and the beliefs that empiricism is equivalent to experimentalism, that experimentation is coextensive with research, that testing a theory is a purely empirical, practical enterprise, and that only what is directly observable and measurable is a legitimate subject for scientific investigation.[10]

The last is particularly relevant here. In the fields of measurement and psychometrics, Michell[11-15] has revealed how and why 'scientific' psychology has misunderstood and distorted the concept of measurement, inventing its own version, and, in the process, abandoning the requirements of empiricism and the canons of science. Michell diagnoses a 'particularly pernicious form of Pythagoreanism'[12] which has led armies of 'scientific' psychologists, operating under the influence of the 'quantitative imperative' (the belief that measurement is a necessary condition of science), into the widespread, blatantly *unscientific*, practice of treating many variables of interest as if they were quantitative, without first doing the scientific job of testing the hypothesis that they are. Thus, psychology's treatment of the concept of measurement evidences 'methodological thought disorder', and a systematic breakdown in its application of scientific method. Even more worryingly, the way measurement and psychometrics are currently taught in the academic institutions 'actually subverts the scientific method' (p. 211).[15] This core problem is exacerbated by additional methodological and statistical confusions in the experimental and data-analytic practices of mainstream psychology.[16-21] Prominent among these is the elision of potentially important individual differences via the use of statistical models in which those differences are conflated with 'random error'.[22]

In mainstream psychology, then, it is not *science*, but a package of distortions driven by *scientism*, by what Chomsky called 'a kind of play acting at science' (p. 559),[23] that prevails. As Bickhard concludes: 'The damaging effect of these mythologies on the process of the science of psychology are multiple and serious. They result in an enormous waste of resources in the pursuit of fallacious notions of how to do "good science" and in the avoidance of and ignorance of scientifically more fruitful alternatives' (p. 322).[10]

It is hardly surprising that scientific psychology is left vulnerable to attack, especially from the non-mainstream postmodernist (a term I use loosely and generically here), who has stepped in to offer a 'new' vision, involving a radical move away from realism and objectivism. This vision is a response to the perceived 'waning of empiricist foundationalism' (p. 13),[24] the failure of scientific observation to guarantee truth and indubitability, the distortions of science's 'ideology of objectivity', the sterility of the outmoded 'Rhetoric of Scientific Truth' (p. 187),[25] and the need for new directions – social constructionism, phenomenology, hermeneutics, ideology critique, and so on.

Indeed, only such movements, it is claimed, are properly equipped to handle the world of *meaning* – a 'plurivocal' world which is infinitely complex, intrinsically elusive, perpetually shifting, necessarily subjective, relativist and value-laden – hence, not surprisingly, excluded by science. In the field of psychological practice, the new 'meaning-making' approaches in psycho-therapy[26] have joined the challenge to traditional ontological and epistemo-logical realism. Even though these approaches are often claimed to be extensions of the 'cognitive turn' (which was always part of the post-beha-viourist scientific mainstream), and even though cognitive therapists may argue that their focus is on the 'development of dysfunctional meaning structures' (p. 12),[27] they typically take cognitions beyond their putatively scientific location, into a constructivist meta-theory which cannot be anything but radically opposed to traditional science,[28] and which is in any case the inevitable outcome of the representationism at the heart of the information-processing framework.[29] In psychoanalysis, too, we are told, there is 'a growing consensus that psychoanalysis is an inherently dialectical discipline that works in an intersubjective field that cannot be fully objectified' (p. 1048).[30]

Consistent with this trend, the recent reinvigoration of qualitative research methods in psychology is hijacked by these ideological commitments; the qualitative/quantitative distinction is mistakenly perceived to be a philo-sophical, rather than an empirical, one;[31,32] and the qualitative resurgence is held to vindicate the rejection of traditional science, whose commitment to the quantitative imperative leaves it unable or unwilling to deal with manifestly non-quantitative variables such as meaning.

These debilitating misconceptions hamper the progress of psychology. What is needed is reconsideration both of science and of meaning, which would reveal that meaning is properly located within the domain of science, and necessarily within scientific psychology, and that a scientific investigation of meaning is well within reach.

The meaning of science

The fashion of the day is to assert that 'any claim to know what science *really* is, is born of arrogance and presumption' (quote by Goldberg, p. 1002).[33] In a climate which Stove[34,35] has aptly dubbed the 'jazz age in the philosophy of science', heralded by Popper,[36,37] popularised by Kuhn[38] and taken up in Bloor's[39] 'strong programme in the sociology of knowledge', conflation of the sociology with the logic of science has become almost dogma. According to Sturdee, science is 'fundamentally a human social activity – there is no such abstract entity ("science") to which we can appeal when shortcomings in the practice of science are identified, allowing us to claim that the problems exist with human activities and not with "science" itself. Actual practice is all there is' (p. 69).[40]

Regardless of 'jazz age' pronouncements, history attests that science has always been a *cognitive* enterprise (but *not* thereby an *unmotivated* one), founded on the assumptions of realism, naturalism and determinism, and aiming variously (though not always simultaneously) to discover, describe, understand, explain and predict.[41] There is of course no (oxymoronic) 'abstract entity' which is 'science', nor would any scientist deny the social nature of scientific activity. Nevertheless, the *content* of science, in the sense of the truth or falsity of its claims, is dependent just on the way the world is; the epistemic aspect of science is logically distinct from its social aspect,[42,43] and, in fact, is what renders coherent allusions such as Sturdee's to 'shortcomings in the practice of science', or general claims that the harnessing of science for political, economic and other gains is at odds with its aspirations to objectivity and the disinterested pursuit of truth. Sturdee himself suggests: 'A golden opportunity for vested interests to *use science for other ends* is evident in the current enthusiasm for evidence-based medicine as it develops into a social movement' (p. 69).[40] No sense could be made of such complaints, or indeed of the whole thrust of sociological analyses of scientific activities, if there were no realist, objectivist core to science.

Given that science is a cognitive enterprise undertaken by multiply-motivated creatures, it does *not* traffic in the indubitable, but acknowledges the fallibility of the senses and the likelihood of motivated distortions. Sternberg alludes to one of the beauties of science being its inbuilt openness to self-correction. Here is the answer to the question why we should *care*, why we should *want* to be scientific at all. Science is our best bet, precisely *because* of its self-consciously sceptical core, prompting us carefully and system-atically to employ the best available error-detection mechanisms. With respect to the various *individual* methods, there are notable styles of scientific thinking other than experimentation,[44] but there is really no limit beyond the single core requirement.

> 'There is no God-given scientific method. Scientific methods are empirically determined. Science is the enterprise of trying to find out how natural systems work. The ways of working of natural systems are difficult for us to discern and we are ill-equipped for the task. Scientific methods are premised upon our cognitive fallibility. Only if our ideas are criticised and tested do we stand some chance of eliminating erroneous ones and locating correct answers. The common core to all scientific methods is *critical inquiry*. This is *the fundamental* scientific method.'[14]

Of course, there is nothing particularly esoteric about this; scientific method is merely 'a potentiation of common sense, exercised with a specially firm determination not to persist in error if any exertion of hand or mind can deliver us from it' (p. 59).[45]

However, science's necessary attunement to the nature of the subject matter of inquiry *does* require a more sophisticated conception of causality than is typically understood by mainstream scientific psychologists or rejected by their opponents. Nothing is a cause or an effect in itself; cause and effect are relative not only to each other, but to the complex conditions of events from which they may be conceptually abstracted. Rather than a simple chain, therefore, causality is more accurately conceived as a field or network, so that a cause is only ever a cause *within a certain field*.[46–48] This conception is crucial not only to appreciating the methodological difficulties arising from individual and contextual variation, but also to properly interpreting scientific evidence. For example, while the randomised controlled trial may be widely regarded as providing the 'highest grade of evidence' (p. 4) in psychotherapeutic effectiveness research,[49] nevertheless, to date, such research has been unable to accommodate crucial differences between: experts and non-experts; mixed methods and relatively 'pure' methods; co-morbidly symptomatic clients versus relatively 'pure' clients; short-term versus long-term treatments; and clients who are left more, rather than less, incapacitated by symptom removal.[50] In addition, choice of treatment approach may require the kind of knowledge of aetiology which is not included in formal psychiatric diagnoses as they are used for sample selection in research trials: 'from a psychodynamic standpoint the lack of specificity of psychiatric diagnostic categories renders them largely uninformative. A diagnosis of anxiety may be no more meaningful to a psychodynamic therapist than a diagnosis of chest pain to a respiratory physician or stomach pain to a gastroenterologist. These would not be regarded as diagnostic categories, so much as symptoms of any number of possible underlying disorders' (p. 167).[50] The same would apply, *mutatis mutandis*, to the central topic of the present book – the concept of, and selection of treatment for, the 'dangerous' person. Thus, unrealistic faith in overly simple causal models is liable to compromise the scientific 'evidence' upon which the psychological intervention of the scientist-practitioner is based.

What follows from all this is a set of conclusions at odds with much current scientistic practice in psychology. Genuine science does not exclude *a priori* any subject matter from its focus of inquiry. Genuine science does not *presuppose* the appropriateness of any individual method (such as measurement), for that must be empirically determined via sensitivity to the nature of the subject matter under investigation. Genuine science does not privilege one kind of variable (say, quantitative) over another kind of variable (say, qualitative). Genuine science does not force its subject matter into uncontextualised linear causal models. These conclusions throw new light onto the possibility of a science of meaning.

The meaning of meaning and its place in scientific psychology

Despite notorious difficulties with the concept of meaning, two categories are initially identifiable: 'linguistic or symbolic' meaning, and 'experiential' meaning.

Linguistic or symbolic meaning usually involves 'referring to', 'signifying', 'standing for', 'indicating', 'substituting for' or 'representing'. This category is further divisible into two kinds. On the one hand are the 'conventional' signs or symbols, such as those which occur in language, mathematical and logical notation, and some social rituals – all of which are determined by convention and learned by the individual in a social setting. On the other hand, 'non-conventional' symbols are those which occur in dreams, symptoms, rituals, myths, art, folklore, etc, and whose meanings are controversial. In both cases 'meaning' is a *three-term relation*, holding between a signifier/symbol, a signified/symbolised, and a person for whom the signifier stands for the signified. Each of these three terms is necessary for any instance of meaning. This relational nature of meaning is an important point about the *logic of meaning*. It follows that meaning cannot be a thing, cannot be intrinsic, cannot be a property, cannot be reduced to just one of the terms, and cannot be converted into a mere binary relation. Many confusions in the literature on meaning are traceable to a failure to appreciate these logical constraints – for example, the collapsing of the signifier and signified, and the obliteration of the signifying subject, in much semiotic and hermeneutic theory. But the most damaging confusion has been the relativisation of the concept of meaning itself, for it is here that constructivism and anti-realism are launched. The fact that, in the meaning relation, each term is related to the other does not imply that there is anything relative about the *existence* either of the entities so related, or of the meaning relation itself. That is, the *fact that x means y to person p* (within such-and-such an environment) is not itself relative – it is a fact as objective and real as any other. For there is nothing inherently mysterious or metaphysical about relations; they are, like any other facts, states of affairs located in the spatio-temporal realm of real events.

Among the logical constraints the most important is that meaning is a relation which requires as one of its terms a *cognising organism*. This brings the field of meaning inextricably into the subject matter of psychology, for it is a point of logic about meaning that every theory of meaning must be a *psychological* theory. Meaning, therefore, is parasitic on *cognition*, which itself may be shown to be not an internal, private state in the Cartesian theatre, but a *two-term relation* between an organism and its environment.[51,52,53] From this logical point, a number of psychological requirements follow, which any general theory of meaning would be expected to meet: the development and selection of meanings; the differences and interrelationships between individual meanings, locally shared meanings and universal meanings; variations in the *tertium comparationis* (what connects the signifier with the signified); and the relationship between conscious and unconscious elements in meaning. In sum, it would be the task of *scientific* psychology to meet systematically the logical constraints and psychological requirements in any theory of meaning. Within this context, a psychologist can begin to investigate the hermeneutic question: *what does x mean to person p?* (e.g. what does Freud represent to the Ratman in the session when the latter cowers in fear in the consulting room?). The general point is that, when these lines of argument are pursued, it becomes clear that the question of meaning, though often difficult, is a perfectly respectable, scientifically amenable one.

The second kind of meaning – 'experiential' or 'existential' meaning, some-times identified as 'personal significance', or the existentialist *Erlebnis* – seems to be somewhat more scientifically intractable. Yet closer scrutiny of the literature reveals that the traditional treatment of this kind of meaning involves unnecessary and misleading mystification. While there is still, loosely speaking, the three terms (person, event, and what that event 'means' to that person), nevertheless, what is at the heart of experiential meaning (e.g. the 'meaning' of my mother's death) is a constellation of beliefs, feelings, motivational states, etc about a particular event or experience. In his critical analysis of the 'meaning-making' movement in contemporary psy-chotherapy, Mackay[28] suggests that this second kind of meaning, which is typically the relevant one in psychotherapy, could more correctly be under-stood to be 'meaning as motivational salience', encompassing both the person's motivational state and the person's beliefs about the relevance of an object or event to the motive. Now here, of course, it becomes clear that what is involved are good old-fashioned psychological states (viz the belief-desire model), and these are perfectly acceptable to scientific psychologists (except radical behaviourists and eliminative materialists). The question of what my mother's death 'means' to me will involve questions such as: what beliefs (conscious and unconscious) do I have about it and about its relation-ship to my needs and wishes; what are those needs and wishes with respect to it; what emotions does it arouse in me; what, perhaps, does it stand for in a symbolic sense? Hence, whether we choose to identify this kind of meaning as what is encapsulated in 'schema-focused' cognitive therapy, or whether we prefer a more psychodynamic formulation, the psychological *categories* involved (beliefs, desires, etc) are the same.

Here, too, meaning is not a property of an event, but a relational phenom-enon, intrinsic neither to the event nor to the person, but just as real and objective as other relations, and 'constructed' only in the sense that it may include false beliefs which are occasionally (misleadingly) described as 'true for me'. Naturally, the investigation of experiential meaning is a difficult and complex enterprise. But complexity is not a criterion for exclusion from scientific investigation. Nor, however complex, do such meanings require any special, mysterious, non-natural processes or realms outside those covered by the ordinary categories of psychological science. This remains true even when, as often happens, the two kinds of meaning, the linguistic/symbolic and the experiential, are found intertwined in complex ways.

As for the view that science deals with causes and not with meanings, that is just another part of the scientistic package of mainstream psychology, encouraged perhaps by the notorious contrast in philosophy between *reasons* and *causes*. Here, again, there are confusions. Examples typically used to illustrate the reason/cause distinction betray a failure to allow causal efficacy to psychological categories (a flat tyre might be the *cause* of or the *reason* for my lateness, but my reluctance to come would always be a *reason*). Yet, once this confusion is dispelled, then reasons, as Sherwood points out, are either identified with causes, or, when contrasted with causes, turn out to be 'those causally relevant factors which become causally relevant precisely because they are taken into consideration, or responded to, by the individual' (p. 160).[54] Thus, meanings and reasons both require cognition, and since only cognising organisms, by definition, enter into cognitive relations, only they can enter into meaning and reason relations. In the case of meanings, the hermeneutic question 'what does x *mean* to person p?' is *different* from the causal questions '*why* does x mean y to person p?' or 'what is the *effect* of x's meaning y to person p?'. Yet this collection of questions illustrates the fact that causal and hermeneutic questions are logically compatible, and that meanings (being states of affairs) may stand as either causes or effects just as may any other state of affairs. Therefore, a science which investigates human behaviour must address questions of meaning and reasons, because those relations are central to its subject matter; psychology requires reference to all three: meanings, reasons and causes.

The return of the science of meaning into mainstream psychology

Given that current conceptions in psychology of the scope and methods of science are inadequate in the ways indicated, what of those approaches, such as psychoanalysis, which explicitly attempt to combine science and meaning, but which have been neglected or marginalised by the mainstream? If it is indeed *scientism*, rather than genuine science, which prevails, then the widespread dismissal of psychoanalysis on grounds of its alleged unscientific nature begins to seem a little ironic.

In fact, I would argue that Freud's psychoanalytic theory – at least, one particular version of it[55] – is an approach which does not share mainstream psychology's scientistic misconceptions of science and of meaning. Instead, it follows in the realist, materialist, Aristotelian/Darwinian biological tradition,[56] thereby having successfully avoided the plague of modern psychology, the Cartesian legacy of a no-win choice between the extremes of idealism and behaviourism. As such, it has a more sophisticated appreciation of the concept of measurement than does mainstream psychology, recognising not only the proper limits of quantification,[57] but also that neither cognition nor meaning is fundamentally quantitative. The theory embraces the compatibility of hermeneutic and causal (including reason) explanation, and it investigates both the 'linguistic/symbolic' and the 'experiential' kinds of meaning. With respect to the former, psychoanalysis is the only psychological theory which has anything substantial and systematic to say about nonconventional meaning, it is the only theory which appreciates the logic of meaning as a relation and meets the resulting psychological requirements, and it is the only psychological theory which gives due recognition to the third term of the meaning relation, the person. Furthermore, it appropriately anchors the study of meanings in the context of a general psychological theory of an *organic signifying subject*,[58] a theory which therefore cannot be detached from developments in biology and the brain sciences.[59]

The recent re-marriage of psychoanalysis and neuroscience is therefore a promising sign. In a political sense, this may serve as a wake-up call to mainstream psychology, which regards neuroscience as the epitome of a scientific approach and psychoanalysis as the epitome of a *pseudo*-scientific approach. But the real value of the combination lies in its conceptual and methodological fruits. At the *First International Neuro-Psychoanalysis Conference* held in London in 2000, which was devoted to the topic of emotion, Oliver Sacks called for 'a neuroscience of the whole person, but also a science of personal meanings'. Others (e.g., Panksepp, Watt, Damasio) appealed to the earlier 'nonreductive neurology' of Luria, and discussed contemporary research into the various neurobiological underpinnings of central psychoanalytic concepts such as instinctual drives, the pleasure and reality principles, attachment, the unconscious, dreams, and defence. Damasio pointed out that his field, until very recently, had simply neglected psychoanalysis, just as it had also neglected the topics of emotion and consciousness – bad topics for science precisely because they involve subjectivity, which was thought to be beyond science's reach. However, in the last couple of decades, as neuroscience has been inching away from a myopic focus on an isolated cortex, consciousness and emotion have begun to take centre stage, along with an evolutionary perspective, an organismic view of human mental functioning, and the importance of homeostasis. Hence, a return to Freud is inevitable, since these were also his central themes.

These developments are part of a number of new overlapping 'revolutions' which are currently sweeping through mainstream psychology – the 'consciousness' revolution, the 'renewed cognitive' revolution, the 'affective' revolution, even the 'meaning' revolution.[59–62] They are characterised by a more holistic, integrative approach which is beginning, finally, to take seriously the fundamental connections between behaviour (itself inescapably cognitive insofar as it is distinguished from mere movement),[52,48] the 'cold' cognition of cognitive experimentalists, and the (often unconscious) 'hot' environment of body and emotion. Here, many psychoanalytic ideas are being revived, albeit typically accompanied by careful avoidance of their grounding in psychoanalytic theory. Psychological practice is also being caught up in these trends. Even in mainstream cognitive behavioural forms of psychological intervention, the role of the body, emotion and 'hot' cognition, including the conflicted, dynamic unconscious and such phenomena as resistance, ambivalence, transference and countertransference, are increasingly becoming acknowledged,[63,64] although therapists still tend to be ill-prepared to deal with them, because their roots in psychodynamic theory have left them marginalised by the knee-jerk mainstream rejection of anything which has obvious connections with Freud.

Evolving techniques in the scientific investigation of meaning

In the past, psychoanalytic and other meaning-focused approaches have suffered from their reliance on methods which have not always adhered to the core scientific requirement of public accessibility and scrutiny. There is some truth in Grünbaum's[65] critique of the psychoanalytic clinical method, and in Spence's criticisms of the traditional ways of reporting case studies: 'It is more than a little ironic that the one profession that knows in such detail the ways in which memory can be deceived should be the one that relies so heavily on unaided recall in its clinical reports' (p. 43).[66]

However, in her discussion of the possibility of a science of experience, Valentine reminds us of the important, but often overlooked, point that 'there is usually public evidence for "private" mental states, in the form of verbal reports, behavioural data or neurophysiological indices' (p. 537).[67] We are now witnessing the rapid development of increasingly refined tools and techniques for corroborating hypothesised aspects of human behaviour which had previously been considered intractable, such as the unconscious beliefs, wishes and emotions which are the components of 'experiential meanings'.[60,61]

For example, the audio-visual recording techniques of the past have progressed to such an extent that today 'frame-by-frame analyses can be made of videotaped facial expressions, gestures and the like. Muscle patterns in the face can be reliably detected and coded to indicate emotions. Tone of voice can be quantified. Sophisticated psycholinguistic analysis of word choice can be made' (p. 163).[57] Such techniques have led to significant work on aspects of 'intersubjectivity' and 'communicative musicality' in the pre-verbal world of the infant.[68-71] And the recently developed Linguistic Intergroup Bias (LIB)[72,73] is a reliable method of identifying unconscious prejudice and bias without the obvious drawbacks of existing 'explicit' questionnaire methods. Neuroscientific imaging techniques are also improving so rapidly that correlational data, properly interpreted, can provide support for claims about psychological processes. According to Kandel, 'we face the interesting possibility that as brain imaging techniques improve, these techniques might be useful not only for diagnosing various neurotic illnesses but also for monitoring the progress of psychotherapy'.[74] In particular, interpersonal processes within the psychotherapeutic relationship, including intuition, empathy, and so-called 'moments of meaning' captured via sensitivity to 'mutative metaphors',[75,76] which may not be *consciously* perceived, nor even require conscious access for their therapeutic effectiveness, may soon be shown to have empirically verifiable foundations in neurophysiological and other bodily processes,[77] and thus be elevated from their lowly status as mere constructions or figments of the psychotherapist's imagination.

Even in the cognitive domain there is increasing acceptance that investigative techniques must take the *body* into account. Thus, as Bucci points out: 'Cognitive scientists today have moved away from their initial reliance on laboratory experimentation and computer modelling to a recognition that most complex mental functions (at least those carried out by protoplasmic information processors rather than transistorised ones) need to be studied in naturalistic or quasi-naturalistic contexts' (p. 995).[33] Bucci goes on to mention a number of different qualitative methods, focusing on their *systematic* nature, and appealing to the well-known concept of 'triangulation', which uses converging data from multiple sources. The fruitful combination of clinical, cognitive and neurophysiological methods is illustrated in Solms's[78] work on dreaming, or in the research of Shevrin and others[79] on the relationships between conscious and unconscious cognitive and affective processes.

All this is not to imply that there are no serious conceptual or methodological issues still to be resolved. It is only to suggest that, once we clarify the meaning of meaning and its place in science, it becomes obvious that specific techniques for its investigation are not beyond the reach of scientific psychology.

Implications for the scientist-practitioner model of treatment

These arguments have important implications both for developing criteria for scientific practice in psychology, and for practitioner training programmes. In his letter, Sternberg emphasises three aspects of the scientist-practitioner model: that 'science informs practice but practice also informs science'; that 'trainees have training in empirically supported procedures'; and that 'competent practising psychologists keep up on the science of psychology'. As things presently stand, the vast majority of practising psychologists are trained within academic institutions, while psychoanalysts are trained in splendid isolation from them. Neither situation is scientifically healthy, although for different reasons.

In the case of the universities, postgraduate training programmes, following mainstream attitudes, tend to pay scant attention to conceptual or historical issues in psychology, dismissing them as 'irrelevant' to practical concerns. Everything I have said about science and meaning applies here – the whole package of confusions is propagated through the training programmes, so that psychologists move into the practical arena armed with various conceptions (or, as I have argued, *mis*conceptions) about the nature and methods of science, including its putatively legitimate exclusion of meaning. The result is either complacent ignorance, or frustrated disenchantment with the narrowness and inflexibility of formal preparation, whose inadequacy for the unexpectedly complex and challenging life forms of the 'real world' is keenly felt.

In the case of psychoanalysis, on the other hand, the lack of contact with universities and other research communities threatens to foster a cult-like, defensive ideology which insulates itself from the core of science – critical inquiry – and from exposure to competing approaches and relevant empirical research methods. Kandel suggests that the institutional problem of psychoanalysis requires a kind of Flexner report, and that 'the psychoanalytic institutes themselves must change from being vocational schools – guilds, as it were – to being centres of research and scholarship' (p. 521).[74] However, any recommendation for institutional co-operation would be worth taking seriously only *if* the necessary changes were to take place in mainstream academic psychology, so that psychoanalysts might then be furnished with an *appropriate* model of scientific research and scholarship.

Such changes would have numerous positive consequences for training in accordance with the scientist-practitioner model, but three in particular are worth highlighting.

First, adopting the more sophisticated conception of causality would result in better handling of the relationship between scientific theory and scientific practice. Although theory and practice appear to have different central aims, the one to discover facts, the other to bring about change (via attempting to apply those facts), the practical question is a species of scientific question. The scientific theory underpinning practice must include: (i) a general theory of human behaviour – the underlying 'theoretical model', from which the treatment predictions are derived; (ii) a theory about 'what works', that is, a theory about the cause–effect relationships between different aspects of intervention and different outcomes; and (iii) a theory which *contextualises* the 'what works', by providing the *how, why* and *under what conditions* it does so. Therefore, attempts to promote the instrumentalist 'it works' approach as separable from theory overlook the role of (iii) in addressing the inevitable gap between (i) and (ii). Therapeutic efficacy (or otherwise) does not entail (or even confirm) the truth (or otherwise) of the theoretical model, and vice versa. To believe that it does so leads to false claims regarding the scientific status of the theoretical models and of the evidence for them. Too often, premature judgements of 'it works' (or 'nothing works') are made when the logic of the connections between these three theoretical aspects, and their relationship to evidence, is misunderstood. Under these conditions, if, for example, research were to suggest (as it seems to) that therapeutic efficacy is largely independent of the particular theoretical model espoused by the therapist, then the scientific practitioner would be concerned to investigate what factors it *does* depend on, and to develop a theory which would account for it. As a result, it may turn out that the efficacy or failure of one type of treatment, derived from one particular theoretical model, is actually best explained by a different theoretical model, or that a particular theoretical model would predict that, under certain conditions, treatments derived from that model are likely to fail. Thus, adopting the more sophisticated conception of causality would lead simultaneously to a recognition of the importance of familiarity with all theoretical models, and to a healthy appreciation of the minefield that is psychotherapeutic outcome research.

Second, understanding the meaning of meaning and its place in science would begin to break down some of the pseudo-boundaries between behavioural, cognitive behavioural, psychodynamic and other theories and treatment models, hence providing theoretical support for changes which are typically proposed from the practical direction. The fact that meaning depends on cognition, and that it involves the basic psychological categories of beliefs and desires, reveals that all psychological models are actually built on the same fundamental components. It explains why behaviourism was eventually forced to recognise the intimate connection between behaviour and cognition, why cognitive-behaviourism, in turn, is being forced to recognise its intimate connection with motivation and emotion, and why the various forms of narrative and constructivist approach must sooner or later acknowledge that they too are dealing with beliefs and desires. At the same time, the genuine sources of divergence among the theoretical models would be more clearly appreciated and addressed; the disputes are about the *specific content* of beliefs, the *particular sources* of motivation, the *connections* between these, and the *relative weighting* given to their status as conscious or unconscious.

Third, appreciating the scientific method as containing the core principle of critical inquiry would see an overhauling of understanding and teaching in the entire field of research methods. When these are finally driven by genuine science, not only would quantitative and qualitative perspectives be recognised to be equally scientifically legitimate, but the choice of which method to adopt would be accurately perceived to be an empirical, rather than an ideological, matter. Because this would require training in *all* forms of research method, it would also equip the scientist-practitioner with the means of critically evaluating the research of others, including claims about 'empirically supported procedures' and the 'best available evidence' in treatment research. Given that the attunement of method to subject matter is required by the nature of science and of the scientific attitude of critical inquiry, this would find its practical parallel for the scientist-practitioner in the attunement of psychological treatment to the particular person/problem/ environment constellation.

Conclusion

The three points which I have just highlighted converge onto my conclusion. For too long, psychology has succumbed either to the irresistible Scylla of mainstream scientism or to the seductive Charybdis of anti-science. The recent integrative trends in psychology which are beginning to embrace the concept of meaning are presently showing signs of being lured into the latter – into irrationalist and relativist philosophies and metatheoretical perspectives. This is hardly surprising, since the only visible model of science is the narrow, distorted, scientistic one. The greatest danger for psychology today is the failure to separate genuine science from misconceptions and distortions born of scientism. And the greatest danger for psychological *practice* is likewise either to be held in thrall by narrow scientism or to misguidedly turn to post-Kuhnian anti-science. The only solution to this dilemma is to expose and correct psychology's misconceptions, and to ground the model of the scientist-practitioner more firmly in genuine science. This would not only vindicate its centre-stage position, but also, in combination with the new integrative trends in psychology, would provide scientific underpinning for the promotion of more flexible, multidisciplinary, multifocal treatment approaches. Whether or not calls for such moves may be justified on political, economic or social grounds, they are certainly justified on scientific grounds.

Acknowledgements

This chapter is based on an invited keynote address delivered at the Annual Meeting of the Danish Psychological Association in Odense, Denmark, March 2001. I am grateful to Roal Ulrichsen and Pierre Laraignou, and to the Danish Psychological Association for their financial support. Preparation of the present version was supported by the Federal Government of Australia through an Australian Research Council Large Grant for 2001–2003. My thanks also to my research assistant, Sean Coward.

References

1 Sternberg R (2003) Email distributed to Division 2 APA members, 5 March 2003, in response to Tavris C (2003) Mind games: psychological warfare between therapists and scientists. *The Chronicle of Higher Education.* **Feb 28.**

2   Eysenck HJ (1985) *Decline and Fall of the Freudian Empire*. Viking Penguin Books, Middlesex (italics in original).

3   Petocz A (2001) Psychology in the twenty-first century: closing the gap between science and the symbol. In: J Morss, N Stephenson and H van Rappard (eds) *Theoretical Issues in Psychology*. Kluwer Academic Publishers, Norwell, MA.

4   Wittgenstein L (1953/1958) *Philosophical Investigations* (trans. GEM Anscombe). Blackwell, Oxford (italics in original).

5   Friedman M (1991) The re-evaluation of logical positivism. *Journal of Philosophy*. **88**: 505–19.

6   Friedman M (1999) *Reconsidering Logical Positivism*. Cambridge University Press, Cambridge.

7   Hibberd FJ (2001) Social constructionism, logical positivism and the continuity of error. Part 1: Conventionalism. *Theory & Psychology*. **11**: 297–321.

8   Hibberd FJ (2001) Social constructionism, logical positivism and the continuity of error. Part 2: Meaning as use. *Theory & Psychology*. **11**: 323–46.

9   Green CD (1992) Of immortal mythological beasts. *Theory & Psychology*. **2**(3): 291–320.

10 Bickhard MH (1992) Myths of science. Misconceptions of science in contemporary psychology. *Theory & Psychology*. **2**(3): 321–37.

11 Michell J (1997) Quantitative science and the definition of 'measurement' in psychology. *British Journal of Psychology*. **88**: 355–83.

12 Michell J (1999) *Measurement in Psychology*. Cambridge University Press, Cambridge.

13 Michell J (2000) Normal science, pathological science, and psychometrics. *Theory & Psychology*. **10**: 639–67.

14 Michell J (2000) *Measurement in Psychology: difficulties and solutions*. Invited address to the Annual Conference, Division of Health Psychology, The British Psychological Society, 6 September 2000, University of Kent, Canterbury.

15 Michell J (2001) Teaching and misteaching measurement in psychology. *Australian Psychologist*. **36**(3): 211–17.

16 Rosnow RL and Rosenthal R (1989) Statistical procedures and the justification of knowledge in psychological science. *American Psychologist*. **44**: 1276–84.

17 Zuckerman M, Hodgins HS, Zuckerman A *et al.* (1993) Contemporary issues in the analysis of data: a survey of 551 psychologists. *Psychological Science*. **4**: 49–53.

18 Gigerenzer G (1987) Probabilistic thinking and the flight from subjectivity. In: L Krüger, LJ Daston and M Heidelberger (eds) *The Probabilistic Revolution*. MIT Press, Cambridge, MA.

19 Grayson DA (1988) Limitation on the use of scales in psychiatry. *Australian & New Zealand Journal of Psychiatry*. **22**: 99–108.

20 Grayson DA (1998) The frequentist façade and the flight from evidential inference. *British Journal of Psychology*. **83**: 325–45.

21 Grayson DA, Pattison PI and Robins G (1997) Evidence, belief and the 'rejection' of the significance test. *Australian Journal of Psychology*. **49**: 64–70.

22 Grayson DA (2003) *Aggregation, quantitative relationships and science in psychology*. Manuscript in preparation.

23 Chomsky N (1959) A review of BF Skinner's *Verbal Behavior*. Reprinted in: JA Fodor and JJ Katz (eds) (1964) *The Structure of Language*. Prentice-Hall, New Jersey.

24 Gergen KJ (1991) Emerging challenges for theory and psychology. *Theory & Psychology*. **1**(1): 13–35.

25 Ibañez T (1991) Social psychology and the rhetoric of truth. *Theory & Psychology*. **1**(2): 187–201.

26 Neimeyer RA and Raskin JD (eds) (2000) *Constructions of Disorder: meaning-making frameworks for psychotherapy*. American Psychological Association, Washington, DC.

27 Perris C (1988) The foundations of cognitive therapy. In: C Perris, I Blackburn and H Perris (eds) *Cognitive Psychotherapy: theory and practice*. Springer-Verlag, Berlin.

28 Mackay N (in press) Psychotherapy and the idea of meaning. *Theory & Psychology*.

29 Maze JR (1991) Representationism, realism and the redundancy of mentalese. *Theory & Psychology*. **1**(2): 163–85.

30 Strenger C (1998) Review of RR Holt (ed.) *Psychoanalysis and the Philosophy of Science. Collected papers of Benjamin B Rubinstein*. International Universities Press, Madison, CT. *International Journal of Psychoanalysis*. **79**(5): 1046–9.

31 Denzin NK and Lincoln YS (1994) *Handbook of Qualitative Research*. Sage, Thousand Oaks, CA.

32 Richardson JTE (ed.) (1996) *Handbook of Qualitative Research Methods*. BPS Books, Leicester.

33 Shevrin H (1995) Is psychoanalysis one science, two sciences, or no science at all? A discourse among friendly antagonists. *Journal of the American Psychoanalytic Association*. **43**(4): 963–1049.

34 Stove DC (1982) *Popper and After: four modern irrationalists*. Pergamon Press, Oxford. Republished (1998) as *Anything Goes: Origins of the Cult of Scientific Irrationalism*. Macleay Press, Sydney.

35 Stove DC (1991) Cole Porter and Karl Popper: the Jazz Age in the Philosophy of Science. In: *The Plato Cult*. Basil Blackwell, Oxford.

36 Popper KR (1959) *The Logic of Scientific Discovery*. Hutchinson, London.

37 Popper KR (1957/1963) *Conjectures and Refutations: the growth of scientific knowledge*. Routledge & Kegan Paul, London.

38 Kuhn T (1962) *The Structure of Scientific Revolutions*. University of Chicago Press, Chicago.

39 Bloor D (1976/1991) *Knowledge and Social Imagery*. Routledge & Kegan Paul, London.

40 Sturdee P (2001) Evidence, influence or evaluation? Fact and value in clinical science. In: C Mace, S Moorey and B Roberts (eds) *Evidence in the Psychological Therapies*. Brunner-Routledge, East Sussex (italics mine).

41 McMullin E (1984) The goals of natural science. Presidential Address delivered before the Eighty-second Annual Western Division Meeting of the American Philosophical Association, Cincinnati, Ohio, April 27. In: *Proceedings and Addresses of the American Philosophical Association*. **58**: 37–64.

42 Friedman M (1998) On the sociology of scientific knowledge and its philosophical agenda. *Studies in the History and Philosophy of Science.* **29**: 239–71.

43 Haak S (1996) Science as social – yes and no. In: LH Nelson and J Nelson (eds) *Feminism, Science and the Philosophy of Science.* Kluwer Academic Publishers, Dordrecht.

44 Crombie AC (1994) *Styles of Scientific Thinking in the European Tradition.* Duckworth, London.

45 Medawar PB (1969) *Induction and Intuition in Scientific Thought.* Methuen & Co. Ltd, London.

46 Anderson J (1938) The problem of causality. In: *Studies in Empirical Philosophy.* Angus & Robertson, Sydney (1962).

47 Mackie JL (1974) *The Cement of the Universe: a study of causation.* Clarendon Press, Oxford.

48 Dretske F (1988) *Explaining Behavior: reasons in a world of causes.* MIT Press, Cambridge, MA.

49 Mace C, Moorey S and Roberts B (2001) *Evidence in the Psychological Therapies.* Brunner-Routledge, East Sussex.

50 Richardson P (2001) Evidence-based practice and the psychodynamic psychotherapies. In: C Mace, S Moorey and B Roberts (eds) *Evidence in the Psychological Therapies.* Brunner-Routledge, East Sussex.

51 Anderson J (1927) The knower and the known. In: *Studies in Empirical Philosophy.* Angus & Robertson, Sydney (1962).

52 Maze JR (1983) *The Meaning of Behaviour.* George Allen & Unwin, London.

53 Michell J (1988) Maze's direct realism and the character of cognition. *Australian Journal of Psychology.* **40**: 227–49.

54 Sherwood M (1969) *The Logic of Explanation in Psychoanalysis.* Academic Press, New York.

55 Petocz A (1999) *Freud, Psychoanalysis and Symbolism.* Cambridge University Press, Cambridge.

56 Hopkins J (in press) Conscience and conflict: Darwin, Freud, and the origins of human aggression. In: D Evans and P Cruse (eds) *Emotion, Evolution, and Rationality.* Oxford University Press, Oxford.

57 Bellack L (1993) *Psychoanalysis as a Science.* Allyn and Bacon, Boston, MA.

58 Kristeva J (1973) The system and the speaking subject. In: The tell-tale sign: a survey of semiotics II. *Times Literary Supplement.* **12 Oct**: 1249–50.

59 Panksepp J (1998) *Affective Neuroscience: the foundations of human and animal emotions.* Oxford University Press, New York.

60 Westen D (1998) The scientific legacy of Sigmund Freud: toward a psychodynamically informed psychological science. *Psychological Bulletin.* **124**(3): 333–71.

61 Westen D (1999) The scientific status of unconscious processes: is Freud really dead? *Journal of the American Psychoanalytic Association.* **47**(4): 1061–106.

62 Damasio A (2000) *The Feeling of What Happens. Body, emotion and the making of consciousness.* Vintage, London.

63 Allison D and Denman C (2001) Comparing models in cognitive therapy and cognitive analytic therapy. In: C Mace, S Moorey and B Roberts (eds) *Evidence in the Psychological Therapies*. Brunner-Routledge, East Sussex.

64 Arkowitz H (2003) Towards an integrative perspective on resistance to change. *Journal of Clinical Psychology*. **58**: 219–27.

65 Grünbaum A (1993) *Validation in the clinical theory of psychoanalysis*. International Universities Press, Madison, CT.

66 Spence D (1993) Traditional case studies and prescriptions for improving them. In: NE Miller, L Luborsky, JP Barber *et al.* (eds) *Psychodynamic Treatment Research*. Basic Books, New York.

67 Valentine ER (1999) The possibility of a science of experience: an examination of some conceptual problems facing the study of consciousness. *British Journal of Psychology*. **90**: 535–42.

68 Malloch S (1999/2000) Mothers and infants and communicative musicality. *Musicae Scientiae: Rhythm, Musical Narrative and Origins of Human Communication*. Special Issue: 29–58.

69 Trevarthen C (1998) The concept and foundations of infant intersubjectivity. In: S Bråten (ed.) *Intersubjective Communication and Emotion in Early Ontogeny*. Cambridge University Press, Cambridge.

70 Stern DN, Hofer L, Haft W *et al.* (1985) Affect attunement: the sharing of feeling states between mother and infant by means of inter-modal fluency. In: TN Field and N Fox (eds) *Social Perception in Infants*. Ablex Publishing Corporation, Norwood, NJ.

71 Stern DN (2000) Putting time back into our considerations of infant experience: a microdiachronic view. *Infant Mental Health Journal*. **21**(1–2): 21–8.

72 Maass A, Salvi D, Arcuri L *et al.* (1989) Language use in intergroup contexts: the linguistic intergroup bias. *Journal of Personality and Social Psychology*. **57**: 981–93.

73 Maass A, Milesi A, Zabbini S *et al.* (1995) Linguistic intergroup bias: differential expectancies or in-group protection? *Journal of Personality and Social Psychology*. **68**: 116–26.

74 Kandel E (1999) Biology and the future of psychoanalysis: a new intellectual framework for psychiatry revisited. *American Journal of Psychiatry*. **156**(4): 505–24.

75 Cox M and Theilgaard A (1987) *Mutative Metaphors in Psychotherapy: the aeolian mode*. Tavistock, London.

76 Cox M and Theilgaard A (1994) *Shakespeare as Prompter. The amending imagination and the therapeutic process*. Jessica Kingsley Publishers, London.

77 Ramachandran VS and Hubbard EM (2001) Synaesthesia: a window into perception, thought and language. *Journal of Consciousness Studies*. **8**(12): 2–34.

78 Solms M (1997) *The Neuropsychology of Dreams: a clinico-anatomical study*. Lawrence Erlbaum Associates, Mahwah, NJ.

79 Shevrin H, Bond JA, Brakel LA *et al.* (1996) *Conscious and Unconscious Processes: psychodynamic, cognitive, and neurophysiological convergences*. Guilford Press, New York.

Chapter 4

Psychopathy: the dominant paradigm

Mark Morris

Within the psychodynamic therapies, there is always a difficult interface with approaches that take a more diagnostic approach. Where a cognitive therapist might diagnose an insect monophobia for someone frightened of spiders, or a psychiatrist make a diagnosis of depression, for the psychodynamic therapist these different classifications do not impart much information. This may be because the cognitive therapist has a different treatment regimen for the different diagnostic groups, as will the psychiatrist. For the psychodynamic therapist, the treatment is usually the same, and the focus is trying to understand, rather than to treat and remove the symptom.

Given this relative disinterest in diagnostic categories, the question arises, why should there be a specific chapter in this volume about a diagnostic group, namely psychopaths? From a psychodynamic perspective, each of us have our psychopathic aspects that benefit from therapeutic scrutiny. Those serving prison sentences will also have aspects of this trait that may be more developed, that can be explored along with the various other aspects of what defines them.

The reason is that during the 1990s in the UK within criminological circles there was a shared attitude to psychopathic people, first that they were untreatable or became more dangerous with psychological therapy treatment, and second, that as a result of this, Grendon should specifically remove this group from treatment. Because, clinically, there seemed to be no justification for this position, or at least it vastly oversimplified what was a complex and difficult issue, a critique of the prevailing opinion needed to be constructed, a rehearsal of which makes up the substance of this chapter. The debate is somewhat dated now, as the nettle has been grasped by the criminological community – this group will not go away, and have a right to rehabilitative efforts along with offenders who are less psychopathic. A variety of programmes specifically targeted at this group are now being developed such as the Violence Reduction Programme[1] and, in the UK, the Dangerous and Severe Personality Disorder treatment programmes.

The psychopathy concept

There are a variety of accounts of the syndrome that has come to be known as psychopathy. Pinel[2] in the nineteenth century described 'manie sans delerie' – madness without delusions. People who because of what they had done, and because of aspects of their behaviour, were clearly very psychiatrically ill, but who were otherwise normal – not suffering from delusions. This sort of experience will be familiar with those who have worked in prisons. One can meet a prisoner, have a perfectly normal chat about things, even some personal things, judge the person to be apparently completely normal, and then learn that he sadistically murdered his victim, holding them hostage and torturing them over several days. If able to question the individual about the offence, they may talk about it in an everyday way, entirely oblivious to the discord it is causing in you, the interviewer. Clearly, there is something crazy about the person, but they are not mad in the psychiatric sense.

Over the decades, there were various attempts to characterise this particular personality constellation. One of the problems that would emerge is that aspects of the callousness and ruthlessness that were often present could be seen in very successful or brilliant people. This observation led to Henderson's proposal[3] that there were three groups of psychopaths, including one, the 'creative psychopath', that captured this dilemma. The classical clinical description, however, was that from Cleckley,[4] who coined the term 'the mask of sanity' to describe this phenomenon.

In the 1980s, Robert Hare in Canada developed a 20 item checklist based upon this clinical description, with a score of 0, 1 or 2 being scored for the different parameters such as glibness, lack of empathy, violence and so on, giving a score out of a total of 40. The checklist was developed and administered with considerable empirical methodological rigour, such that there is a high degree of correlation between the scores that different raters would independently give to the same person.[5] There are now a large number of studies that demonstrate that the risk of further violent recidivism is predicted by the score on this 'Revised Psychopathy Checklist' – the PCL-R.

The result is that the PCL-R is the gold standard in the prediction of risk. It can be criticised in terms of its 'face validity' – the items can be read as a list of unpleasant attributes about an individual, so that it structures abuse rather than anything else. There is a problem in that it is largely based upon historical data – previous offences and behaviour – so there is an implication that high scorers will always be dangerous, and there is no possibility that they will ever change. In spite of these, its influence continues to grow.

The psychological treatment and rehabilitation of offenders received a considerable setback in the late 1970s and 1980s, following an influential article by Martinson arguing that 'nothing works' for recidivists.[6] Some have argued that the subsequent 'collapse of the rehabilitative ideal' in custodial policy was politically driven disinvestment in rehabilitative work. However, it led in the 1980s and 1990s to focusing on the empirical investigation of the efficacy of psychological programmes, pooled together in meta-analytic studies. The efficacy of some programmes could be demonstrated, and distinguishing the features of these led to the development of the 'What Works' movement in criminal psychology. Along with a strong evidence base, the other characteristics of 'What Works' programmes were the identification of programmes that were ineffective (mainly more psychodynamic ones) and to rigidly set down the contents of the programme to be followed, enforcing local compliance with a heavy audit burden, for example videotaping each session for later review.

The cogent argument behind this regimentation of these programmes was first, that the evidence base was established on a particular curriculum, and that to be effective, the programme delivered needed to follow this. Second, that close auditing might minimise the problem of 'programme drift', which might lead to a deviation from the validated programme. The beneficial spin-off was that resource allocation followed a similarly ordered and regimented approach, and these programmes were successful in arguing for and obtaining resource. The downside was that a rather centralist policy culture developed, with little opportunity for those at the coalface to challenge fundamental assumptions. One of these fundamental assumptions was that people with high PCL-R scores should be excluded from the 'What Works' psychological programmes.

The reasoning for this was sound from one perspective. Cognitive psychological treatments require a positive and trusting therapeutic alliance. The client needs to accept they have a problem, to complete their homework tasks, and generally to work with the programme. On average, those with higher PCL-R scores are likely to be more difficult to bring to the table in this regard. Moreover, given the prevalence of duplicity and manipulation in this group, often when they have come to the table, they don't really mean it, or are delighting in fooling the facilitator with their false engagement. Further concern was raised that even where high PCL-R scorers apparently successfully completed programmes, this was false. Even worse, that high PCL-R scorers who were successful in their programmes might become more dangerous, because they would have learned some psychological and social skills to be able to be better and more effective psychopaths in future.

Criticising the concept

There are four main challenges to this position: that it is unscientific; that it involves a diagnostic category mistake; that it is reactionary; and that it is not clinically borne out.

In his epistemological investigation of the nature of scientific knowledge, Popper was clear to identify psychoanalysis and Marxism as not scientific. He proposed that science was based on the refutation of hypotheses, that for a theory to be scientific the issue was less whether it could be proved, than whether it could be disproved. Science proceeds by the proposal of hypotheses to explain phenomena that are subsequently disproven by subsequent generations. A new hypothesis is proposed to explain the situation and so on.

Neither the hypotheses of Marxism nor those of psychoanalysis can be refuted in this way. If a psychoanalyst suggests a man's chewing of a cigar represents a phallic symbol to hide impotency, and the man denies it, the psychoanalyst may suggest that the denial confirms how anxious about impotence the man is. Likewise, if a worker quite likes working in the factory, this is interpreted as a 'false consciousness'. Really he *is* oppressed; the owner of the factory has just manipulated him into believing he is not. This criticism can be extended to all the interpretative disciplines, so that interpretations, be they psychoanalytic, political or anything else, are merely opinions, and cannot claim the authority of science.

The exclusion of high PCL-R scorers from rehabilitative programmes rests on an interpretation of how the individual will behave. This interpretation can become almost completely irrefutable. If an individual acknowledges his responsibility for his offending and requests a programme, and acknowledges the problem that the psychologist will expect him to lie and dupe, because he has so in the past, this acknowledgement will be interpreted as even more devious manipulation by the psychopath. If the individual tries to challenge his exclusion with the help of his lawyer, this will be further interpreted as devious troublemaking behaviour, likewise if the issue is taken into the courts. At no point is the hypothesis that the individual wishes to engage in the programme for malign and manipulative reasons refutable. As such, the hypothesis is unscientific. The PCL-R score on which the interpretation is based is highly scientific, and the legitimacy of the scientifically derived score is mistakenly carried over into the interpretation of the results.

The evidence base, however, remains sketchy, perhaps because of the exclusion of these groups, so that comparative studies are difficult to do. The most oft quoted study was from the erstwhile Penetanguishene therapeutic community (TC) in Canada. Rice *et al.*[7] found that at follow-up, lower PCL-R scorers had improved, whereas the high scorers had become more dangerous – measured by reconviction. This study has been heavily criticised, both challenging whether it was a TC in the UK sense, and because the treatment was compulsory rather than voluntary, with the possibility of the psychological treatment exacerbating pre-existing problems.

The second criticism of the concept is that it derives from a misapplication of the concept of personality disorder. Personality disorder is a clinical diagnosis that is difficult to operationally define. The psychiatric classificatory manuals detail the different symptom groups that will contribute to the diagnosis of a particular personality. These personality disorder descriptions are best conceived of as personality traits, so that some have a strong borderline trait, some obsessional and some a psychopathic trait. The other way of understanding personality is to look on the different descriptions as personality types.

Either way, understanding psychopathic personality as a type or as a trait, there is nothing to suggest that each person with a psychopathic personality will have all of the characteristics that are listed as possible. The assumption that is made in the psychopathy concept is that a high PCL-R scorer will then by definition have a full house of Cleckley-type psychological symptoms. This assumption is a category mistake. A high PCL-R scorer is simply that – a high PCL-R scorer, and a person with a high risk of recidivism. No inference can be drawn on the basis of the score alone about the characteristics of the individual's personality. The PCL-R is not a clinical diagnostic tool, it is a risk assessment tool. The category mistake is first to assume that a high PCL-R score makes a clinical diagnosis of the personality disorder, and second to assume that the fallacious diagnosis made means that the individual will simplistically have all of the possible symptoms listed in the psychiatric classificatory tables. On the basis of several of the symptoms possessed by some of those with psychopathy, all of those scoring above a certain level are excluded from rehabilitative programmes.

The third criticism of the psychopathy concept is more psychodynamic. Working with offenders is a difficult business. Trying to carry out rehabilitative programmes with them is even more so, because of the unsavoury and disturbing content of their material, and because of the disappointingly high failure rate. The rehabilitative zeal, enthusiasm and stamina of criminologists is to be heartily praised, but it seems to come at a price.

Some of the rhetoric about the high PCL-R scoring offender can sound loaded with hatred and fear. It seems that the high PCL-R scoring group have become the folklore 'bogey men' of criminal justice rehabilitation. Untouchable, untreatable, unable to be rehabilitated in any way, and a minority freely able to be persecuted by being abandoned in prison. Furthermore, the justification for not engaging them in treatment is that to do anything else would (allegedly) make them more dangerous. What may be more dangerous is the assumption that those with lower scores both in prisons and without are very much less dangerous; very much less capable of manipulating and duping.

The final criticism is that, clinically, individuals are individual. While a certain amount can be gleaned from a patient's PCL-R score, by no means does this define them. Some high PCL-R scorers are now ready for and responsive to treatment, and make good progress; some are quite refractory, and repeated efforts at treatment result in the work breaking down in very similar circumstances. While this might be interpreted as them having made no progress, arguably, having survived the struggle of treatment for a period, having learned a little along the way, even if the central vulnerability has not been able to be addressed – this does represent some form of psychological movement, even if not explicit symptomatic improvement.

A psychodynamic approach to psychopathy

This attempt to deconstruct some of the practice and folklore that surrounds psychopathy from a psychodynamic perspective does not mean that a psychodynamic approach has no position on the issue. However, broadly, a psychodynamic perspective would not see psychopathy as a personality type, or even particularly as a diagnosis, but rather as a defence. The concept of psychopathy, therefore, describes a defensive psychic structure used to a greater or a lesser extent by all. The high PCL-R scorer has historically demonstrated a number of behaviours that indicate that this psychopathic defence is frequently used, or is a principal defensive strategy for the individual.

A psychodynamic perspective would accept the core psychopathology proposed for the psychopath, namely that there is a lack of an empathetic resonance with the victim. Without an empathetic resonance, there is no inbuilt check to the articulation of aggressive and destructive impulses within a relationship. While it might be rather common among parents to feel like hitting their kids, some empathetic sense that we have of the trauma of being assaulted by an adult in the vulnerable position of being a child stops us from doing it. While we all might at times be tempted by a physically attractive member of the opposite sex, most of us desist from expressing this desire because of an empathetic sense of the trauma of being sexually assaulted, or of the potential trauma within our own partnership. Without this empathetic check on behaviour, the person with a strong psychopathic defensive structure has no internal way of evaluating the trauma that the enactment of his or her wishes will cause.

It is easy to translate this difficulty into a moral and ethical frame. Without an empathetic resonance, the psychopath has no way of conceptualising 'do as you would be done to', because there is no sense of a psychological connection with the other to evaluate how it feels to be 'done to'. Likewise, the 'love thy neighbour as thyself' exhortation cannot connect. The Kantian conclusion that people must be treated as 'ends' rather than 'means' is predicated on an empathetic sense that each person has individual rights. Without the empathetic link, the psychopath does just that – treats everybody that they meet as a means of personal gratification or gain. The notion of the individual as an 'end' in themselves cannot be conceptualised.

This discussion naturally leads onto an account of the developmental process that results in the psychopathic defence becoming predominant. The reason why a psychopath has no conception of the trauma and suffering of the other person is because they have no conception of their own trauma and suffering. The reason for the psychopath having no conception of their own trauma and suffering is because it has been so extreme that the only way to manage it has been to expunge it from their awareness. The psychodynamic hypothesis would be that the psychopathic individual during development has experienced such extreme trauma in the form of physical, sexual, emotional abuse that they develop a method of managing the trauma that they experience. They simply disavow the trauma. They simply learn not to experience the trauma. After a while, by not allowing themselves to experience trauma, they can live and function in the abusive environment more effectively. Psychopathy as a defence is an adaptive strategy to living in intensely traumatic situations.

A similar phenomenon can be seen in the accounts of soldiers in combat. The anxiety about personal safety is difficult; the first kill is difficult; the first near miss or friend killed and dying in agony is difficult, but after a while, killing, people dying and the near misses become simply boring. The psychopathic defence adaptively builds up, such that the effects of intensely traumatising experiences are simply not felt. Likewise, the infliction of intense trauma and cruelty on others is simply not felt. The personal ability to experience emotional trauma is blunted and silenced, and in parallel, the ability to resonate empathetically with the trauma of others fades. In passing, it is interesting to note that a central problem in the post-traumatic difficulties of soldiers who have returned from combat is a sense of guilt. Sometimes in the field, something occurs that collapses the psychopathic defence – a child cries in the same way a sibling used to when frightened – some incident is so terrible that it psychically crashes through the boredom – the psychopathic defence is collapsed, and the soldier is no longer able to function, paralysed by fear and horror as the personal sense of emotional response to trauma and the empathetic resonance returns. In passing, it is interesting to note that often the mutative experience of quite psychopathic people is something that triggers a memory of trauma. Usually there is a screen memory of some extreme trauma – mother with a bloodied face during a fight with father who then turned on the individual, for example – but a memory that is devoid of emotion. Something may happen – either a psychodynamic formulation, or an account from a peer, or some other chance thing – something happens to return the emotion to the memory. The recognition of fear and trauma in the memory can then be extended to the expressions of fear on those that the patient has callously beaten over the years.

Psychopathy as a characteristic defence of some personalities occurs when such extreme trauma has been an everyday developmental experience. The personality forms in a situation where such a defensive structure is required. Psychopaths are people who have grown up in a war zone. As adults, they seek out or create war zones in which their psychopathic defences are again adaptive.

There is a criticism that can be levelled at this model, namely people can develop psychopathic personalities brought up in supportive environments. For example, the high PCL-R scorer adopted at birth into a genuinely loving and supportive family. To understand this paradox, one needs to decouple the two different issues of on the one hand, the reality of trauma, and on the other, the perception of trauma. Normal situations can be experienced as traumatic for some people. There is no objective reason for being afraid of spiders in the UK, but many people are. For a psychopathic defence to form within an individual, all it needs is for their world to feel like a war zone. It does not necessarily need to be one.

Paradoxically, while the psychopaths are perceived as the 'hard men' of popular culture, from a psychodynamic perspective, the opposite may be true. The central pathology of the psychopath may be that they are psychically too vulnerable to the traumas of everyday life and relationships, such that they need to build up a psychopathic defensive shell. Most people can experience the frustrations and trauma of everyday life, and survive them without having to close down our emotional resonance. For the psychopath, these same experiences may be too traumatising. The core pathology of psychopathy may be extreme psychic vulnerability that results in the building of a protective psychopathic unemotional shell. Characteristic of this shell is that the more trauma that is thrown at it, the stronger and harder it becomes. Psychopaths thrive in violent and adversarial situations; these simply make them stronger.

Traditionally, the evidence of genetic transmission of psychopathy or criminality (where the likelihood of a person serving a long prison sentence is greater if a parent or blood relative is doing so) is explained in terms of the inheritance of some sort of hard personality characteristic. A 'psychopathy' gene if you will. A psychodynamic conception might propose that what may be inherited is this extreme emotional vulnerability that requires the development of an unemotional, psychopathic exterior to survive.

A second complication of this account revolves around the notion of vertical splits in the personality. The popular conception of Dr Jekyll and Mr Hyde – a single person with different characteristics – illustrates a reality about personalities, namely that they can comprise different parts; sub-personalities. What is significant about this in relation to psychopathy is that the different sub-personalities will utilise the psychopathic defence to different degrees. A common story is that of a rather meek and timid man who changes into a violent psychopathic individual under the influence of alcohol. Many people are serving long sentences for crimes committed by the psychopathic parts of sub-personalities that they struggle to be aware of, let alone be able to comprehend or integrate in a way that can enable some more control to be exerted.

A second main thrust of a psychodynamic account of psychopathy would be to emphasise that, as a defence, it is ubiquitous to a greater or lesser degree. Everyone has both the ability to develop their psychopathic defence, and everyone functions to some degree psychopathically. The surgeon who needs to close down some of their emotional resonance in order to carry out disfiguring surgery; the mother who goes to work in spite of the children's distress. Often, in more normal settings, the psychopathic defence is employed in the interests of some greater good. The surgery may be life-saving; the mother may need to work for her own mental health or to feed the family. Nevertheless, these would be examples of situations where a psychopathic defence is being used in a normal situation.

The idea that a capacity for psychopathy is endemic may be easy to say, but the implications are a little more difficult to process. From a psychoanalytic perspective, for example, the content of dreams during sleep are driven by wishes. In our dreams and fantasies we are all psychopathic, dreaming about violent or perverse sexual activities, vicariously enjoying the violence of the latest high body count action movie, masquerading our savouring of the details of the latest human tragedy in the news. These avenues are all ways for people to satiate their psychopathic appetites in ways that do not do actual harm to others.

From this perspective, the difference between the high PCL-R scorer and the Joe Public jury member is not that one is psychopathic and the other is not. It is that one has found a means of maintaining his psychopathic tendencies in the realm of fantasy, rather than it spilling over into the real world. One dreams of murder and rape, or watches it in films and on telly. The other actually does it.

One important corollary of this is that it collapses the 'them and us' feel of a lot of the literature about psychopathy. We fool ourselves about our own nature if we believe that we cannot understand the psychopath. We have all wished to do what they have done. We can all understand (if we are honest about ourselves) how and why they have come to act as they have. Psychopaths are not an alien species that we cannot understand. They can be understood, and can be engaged with.

A main psychodynamic contribution to the debate about psychopathy is to undermine the concept as a typology to be studied from a distance, arguing that psychopathy is a question of degree rather than type. Second, it dismantles to some degree the folklore hatred and fear of the minority, arguing that such tendencies are present in the majority, and that the small group of high PCL-R scorers merely represent an extreme end of a statistical bell-shaped distribution within the population.

In some of the debates about psychopathy, concern is expressed that in standard cognitive-didactic offender behaviour programmes, the psychopath will manipulate the sessions, dupe the facilitator into thinking that they are making progress when they are not, and generally present a duplicitous picture. From the psychodynamic perspective, this concern also collapses. For the effective delivery of cognitive-type psychological therapies, there is a need to establish and maintain a positive working alliance. For example, the therapist will give the patient homework that the patient will be required to complete. The therapist will ask questions, and the patient will be expected to answer truthfully. Such an assumption is based upon a medical model where the patient or offender accepts that they have a disease or problem for which they are getting help from the doctor, therapist or expert. In turn, the patient or offender will in good faith put this help into practice. The pathology of the psychopath, it is argued, will interfere with this medical model at all stages. They will not recognise the legitimacy of the expert and will work to undermine it. They will fool the expert into believing that they accept the expert diagnosis, and that they are going along with the prescribed actions, and will take delight in further fooling the therapist into believing that they have made progress, when they have done no such thing.

From a psychodynamic perspective, the good faith of any patient is not assumed. It is central to a psychodynamic understanding of the mind that one part of the mind is constantly lying to other parts of the mind, that lying and deceit are involved in everyday encounters. That good faith and honesty to oneself about oneself are unattainable, let alone good faith and honesty to others. For a psychodynamic treatment, the question is: what is the current state of this faith? To what extent is the patient duping/lying to the therapist today, and why might this be?

In a psychodynamic treatment, the treatment alliance is never assumed. Rather, it is always the central problem, to be observed and explored. From the state of the therapeutic alliance comes valuable information about the nature of object relations, and about previous experience in relations. In short, the psychopath struggles in a medical model cognitive treatment because of the need for a good faith treatment alliance. In a psychodynamic treatment, no such alliance is required. Duplicity is assumed as a starting point, and the task is the exploration of this.

A second corollary of the notion of psychopathic defensiveness being a normal phenomenon is that alongside the need of the surgeon and mother to be psychopathic at times in the interests of the greater good, the defence can be used in the service of less altruistic motives. For example, in all populations, those individuals who are more highly psychopathic will engender fear and hatred borne out of an inability to understand their actions (in the form of crimes); they will engender societal disgust and horror. One way of managing this fear and loathing is to hate, persecute or kill this group, as happens in some jurisdictions. I would argue that the demonisation of this group in the 1990s as part of the 'What Works' movement was itself a psychopathic reaction to the personal and professional challenges that this group represent.

The exclusion of this group from hope of treatment of their problems; their exclusion from opportunities for rehabilitation required a collective shutting down of an empathetic response to how it would feel to be subject to this policy. To be an individual stuck in the double bind of not being able to progress up the rehabilitative ladder towards release without attending offending behaviour programmes on the one hand, but being told that you were excluded from such programmes on the other creates an extreme sense of hopelessness and trauma. To be able to inflict this requires an ability to shut down an empathetic response.

Psychopathy in treatment

The majority of this chapter has been taken up with a critique of some common conceptions of psychopathy, arguing that the pathology can be understood and engaged with in psychological treatment, and looking at some of the reasons why this is difficult. In this discussion, there has been no attempt to propose an alternative programme that might be more successful with this group. Unfortunately, prognosis needs to be guarded about the potential for change.

Some of the treatment initiatives that have been developed have conceptualised the difficulty in terms of various behavioural aspects. For example, the main troubling symptom of the psychopath is their violence, physical and/ or sexual, and this specific symptom might be focused on using a variety of techniques. Such thinking seems to be behind the Violence Reduction Programme, and other initiatives based on this approach. To some extent, this approach may well be successful. If the psychodynamic model of psychopathy as a ubiquitous defence is right, then the only thing that distinguishes me from a long-term high PCL-R prisoner is that I can control my violence and they cannot. There is no need to alter the internal violent cognitions or attitudes if the principal damaging symptom, the violence, can be controlled.

Another approach is to identify the main difficulty in treating this group is their motivation for treatment. The 'responsivity' of a person to treatment is the degree to which the target behaviour is responsive to the programme. Clearly, for psychopaths, there is a problem (apparently) because they are not responsive to the treatments that are offered. It is hoped that psychopaths will be more amenable to treatment courses once they have engaged in a focused piece of motivational interviewing.

The psychodynamic approach does not propose such a programmed intervention. In the variety of settings that psychodynamic treatment takes place, in individual treatment, in groups, and in therapeutic communities, the task is exploration. The task is to explore and understand how and why people are the way they are. To explore and understand the contribution of their experiences, and the meaning of their actions, be they violent or otherwise. There is a belief that if people understand better why they do things, if people can understand themselves better, then they can identify the choices that they have more, and can choose the right things to do, rather than being carried along to do the wrong.

References

1   Wong S (in press) *The Violence Reduction Programme.*
2   Pinel P (1801) *Traite medico-philosophique sur l'alienation mentale ou la manic.* Richard Caille et Ravier, Paris.
3   Henderson D (1939) *Psychopathic States.* WW Norton, New York.
4   Cleckley H (1941) *The Mask of Sanity.* Mosby, St Louis.
5   Hare R (1991) *Manual for the Hare Psychopathy Checklist Revisited.* Multi-health Systems, Toronto.
6   Martinson R (1974) What Works? Questions and answers about prison reform. *The Public Interest.* **10**: 22–54.
7   Rice M, Harris G and Cormier C (1992) An evaluation of a maximum security therapeutic community for psychopaths and other mentally disordered offenders. *Law and Human Behaviour.* **16**: 4.

Chapter 5

Changing people with programmes

Richard Shuker

Interventions with offenders have reflected not only the scientific status of the treatment method but also the prevailing political and social climate. Convicted offenders have been subject to a range of treatment approaches from the 'boot camp' to encounter groups, transactional analysis and supportive counselling. The fluctuating trend between the optimism which facilitated developments in pioneering treatments such as therapeutic communities in the 1960s and the pessimism in offender treatment which was to follow points to the fleeting and tenuous nature of the influence enjoyed by the different therapeutic traditions.

The hope that treatment could provide a rehabilitative function was questioned in a series of studies from North America. These studies had a profound influence on rehabilitation policy and practice. Perhaps the best known of these studies was by Martinson who concluded that, 'with few and isolated exemptions, the rehabilitative efforts that have been reported have had no appreciable effect on recidivism'.[1] Similar conclusions were also reached by other researchers[2,3] and these findings became cited as the 'nothing works' doctrine in the reduction of criminal recidivism.

The 'nothing works' conclusion influenced policy at both ends of the political spectrum, with both the left and right finding evidence to support their beliefs about the disposal of offenders. From this conclusion it could be argued that the causes of crime could justifiably be cited as being outside the individual and being socially determined. However, equally persuasive is the argument that if nothing works then a punishment approach should be stepped up a gear. This 'just deserts' idea evolved into a 'humane containment' model of incarceration and practice became embedded within an uneasy compromise between these positions. The overwhelming consequence of this was to dampen research interest and constrain clinical practice in the field of offender rehabilitation for over 10 years. The 'nothing works' view attained a dogma-like status in the minds of the majority of professionals within the criminal justice system, and its validity was not to become questioned until the 1980s.

The 'nothing works' position became increasingly challenged in both the UK[4,5] and in North America.[6] However, it was developments in the field of statistical analysis, in particular meta-analysis, which gave the growing body of sceptics the real means to present a credible and potent challenge to the prevailing ideological and theoretical stance. The use of meta-analysis to combine different reviews, and tease out trends from different studies where positive outcomes had been indicated, enabled researchers to identify a series of key variables which appeared to be associated with favourable outcome and in particular with a reduction in recidivism. Meta-analytic reviews can be used to evaluate treatments even where the studies included in the review may have been substantially different (for example, differences in design or length of treatment). Any methodological flaws in the studies reviewed can also be controlled for. The conclusions drawn from these reviews made a substantial impact within the field of offender rehabilitation and dictated a major shift in both theory and practice.

The development of a 'psychology of criminal conduct'

One of the most important findings to emerge from the evidence base which surfaced in the 1980s was the notion that interventions could be successful if they adopted certain principles. Three fundamental theoretical assumptions came to underlie rehabilitative practice and became regarded as a 'Psychology of Criminal Conduct' (PCC).[7] This conceptual model has become the basis of the development of the central treatment framework within forensic practice. The principles which appeared most central to successful outcome (in terms of decreased recidivism) were those of risk, need and responsivity. These three principles impacted substantially upon the development of treatment.

The risk principle

The risk principle argues that the treatment offered to offenders should reflect the level of risk presented. This is defined in terms of the largely static historical factors which are predictive of future recidivism. A review of successful interventions[8] indicated that interventions which used risk to assess the level of treatment required (providing higher risk offenders with greater quantity of service and assigning lower risk offenders to more minimal service provision) were more effective in reducing recidivism than those treatments which did not structure and implement treatment on this basis.

The need principle

Perhaps the most influential idea was the concept of criminogenic need. This suggested that certain aspects of an individual's behaviour and lifestyle directly contributed to or were supportive of offending. It suggested that certain offender characteristics were strongly associated with offending and that these should form the direct focus for treatment. Inherent within this principle is the importance of distinguishing between offender problems which are and are not associated with recidivism. Matching the identified criminogenic needs of offenders with the stated aims of the treatment is a concept which has underpinned the development of interventions. Central to the need principle is the idea that criminal conduct is associated with risk factors that are dynamic – that is, they are subject to change, and include areas such as deficits in coping skills, offence supportive beliefs, substance misuse, maladaptive cognitive appraisals, externalisation of responsibility, and poorly developed interpersonal problem-solving skills. The development of interventions for offenders has been strongly influenced by the rationale which suggests that these dynamic risk factors need to form the primary targets for intervention. It also advocates the importance of a systematic and structured assessment of offender needs to ensure they match the goals of intervention. For example, if the identified needs of an offender concern an impulsive and aggressive reaction to the perception of interpersonal threat, there may be little justification in a referral to a vocational training course if deficits in this area are not present.

A criticism of the 'nothing works' literature was that the 'nothing works' conclusion had been drawn from interventions which had targeted aspects of an individual's problems which had little relevance to offending.[9] A scepticism developed towards addressing psychological functioning or mental health needs which were not assumed to be related to recidivism as illustrated succinctly by Andrews: 'If recidivism reflects anti social thinking, don't target self esteem, target anti social thinking' (p. 13).[8] Furthermore, factors regarded as being related to personal distress and '. . . vague emotional complaints . . . whether assessed by way of sociological constructs of anomie, strain and alienation or by way of clinical constructs of low self esteem, anxiety, depression, worry or officially labelled "mental disorder"' are identified as minor or less promising targets for treatment (p. 37).[10] For example, turning somebody into a better person where any definition of better person is not linked to recidivism is regarded as, at best, a less promising target for intervention.[7] Interventions with offenders which sought to alleviate psychological functioning and personal well-being as their primary treatment goal were considered to be driven by a theoretical framework of little relevance to the reduction of recidivism.

The responsivity principle

The third principle underlying the Psychology of Criminal Conduct is that of responsivity. This principle argues that the therapeutic techniques adopted must be matched to the offender's learning style. The clinical techniques used and style of delivery adopted must be those which are able to engage, interest and motivate the participants in order for them to respond. This principle had an important impact at a number of levels. It suggested that if offenders were offered treatment that used techniques which were not compatible with their learning styles, the chances of successful outcome were reduced and, moreover, there was a distinct possibility that treatment could actually lead to increased criminal recidivism.[11] For example, submitting interpersonally anxious offenders to confrontational encounter group therapy may be psychologically damaging to those individuals and is highly unlikely to lead to positive results in the form of reduction in recidivism or otherwise. A consensus of opinion emerged as to the types of treatment style and technique which offenders were most likely to respond to. These included methods such as: '. . . anti criminal modelling, teaching concrete skills . . . for example, role-playing, graduated practice, reinforcement, making resources available, verbal guidance and cognitive restructuring' (p. 421).[12]

A consensus also emerged regarding the treatment methods which offenders did not respond to and within this was a strong scepticism towards interventions not based on the cognitive behavioural model including those:

> '. . . designed according to the principles of clinical sociology, the principles of deterrence and labelling, innovative intermediate punishments, and unstructured psychodynamic therapy'.[10] (p. 56)

The programme approach

An explicit theoretically driven model, supported by empirical evidence of its efficacy in impacting upon recidivism, provided the starting point for differentiating the programme treatment approach from the range of other interventions. The need to establish an empirical evidence base had clear implications for the theoretical models on which treatment became structured.

Psychodynamic approaches

The problems for psychodynamic treatment in establishing an evidence base that was accessible to outside scrutiny and an association with a less unstructured and unfocused mode of delivery virtually excluded the integration of psychodynamic interventions from the mainstream orthodoxy of forensic practice. The prevailing view has come to reflect the conclusions of the meta-analysis by Andrews *et al.*[13] that these approaches tend to *increase* recidivism. The review concluded that: 'Traditional psychodynamic approaches and non directed therapies are to be avoided with general samples of offenders' (p. 377). Psychodynamic approaches became largely marginalised and were regarded as having little of value to offer to the debate about what interventions offered promise.[14]

The cognitive behavioural and social learning perspectives

Social learning theory

Whilst behavioural and learning approaches have provided the basis for understanding the processes by which antisocial behaviour is both learned and maintained, approaches which focus primarily on behaviour modification through the use of reward and punishments have been criticised for having limited ability to promote the generalisation of new behaviours and skills beyond the treatment setting.[15] The development of social learning theory incorporated ideas such as expectations, learning through observation and the functioning of an internal self regulatory system.[16] Within this model, behaviour is seen to be influenced by environmental factors, core beliefs and immediate situational appraisals (for example, a person's value system which dictates that, in a given situation, a perception of being insulted should be responded to by retribution). The social learning model for offender treatment has proved particularly relevant to interventions with violent offenders. Behaviour is modified through targeting the expectations, appraisals, belief systems and reinforcing contingencies associated with violent behaviour.

Cognitive behavioural theory

The role of temperamental, social, familial and environmental factors in the aetiology of criminal behaviour is now not widely disputed. However, the cognitive behavioural paradigm suggests that the factors involved in the *maintenance* of criminal conduct are more *psychological* than social. The perspective that human conduct is determined by cognitions and the belief systems which underpin them has become central to the devolvement of interventions. Andrews[10] suggests that although cognitive and behavioural ideas draw from the psychodynamic formulations such as that of Glueck and Glueck,[17] the major factors of significance to criminal behaviour are cognitive and attitudinal factors. It is these factors which mediate between social, environmental and temperamental determinants and acts of antisocial behaviour. Meta-analytic studies supported this view with substantial evidence that interventions which offered the most promising outcomes are based on the cognitive behavioural approach.[13,18,19]

Cognitive behavioural interventions are based on the psychological principle that cognitive processes affect behaviour and that it is biases in perception and errors in information processing which lead to a range of antisocial and aggressive behaviours. The work of Beck[20] in identifying 'faulty thinking' continues to be influential in focusing treatment on biases in thinking and interpretation. The cognitive behavioural approach suggesting that mental health problems such as anxiety and depression were largely a result of these distortions in thinking became applied to the domain of antisocial behaviour. Core beliefs and attitudes about self and others are formed early in life but continue to exert a major influence on how offenders see the world. For example, Beck[21] considered specific rigid beliefs to be highly instrumental in acts of violence. Beliefs such as authority being controlling and unjust, people being untrustworthy and hostile, and spouses being deceitful and rejecting provide, he suggested, the foundations for the hostile interpretations of the actions of others with the perception of blame fundamental in much of violent behaviour.

This approach argues for three strands to intervention. First, an exploration of hostile or self-serving belief systems by examining the evidence upon which they are based whilst focusing on the development of a more adaptive belief system which allows for an alternative way in which to make sense of the world. Second, a modification of the immediate appraisals, interpretations and thinking styles of offenders in a manner which allows offenders to construct their experiences in a non-threatening, blaming or justifying way. Third, teaching a range of new pro-social behaviours and skills including problem solving, coping and self-management.

Skills-based interventions

The influence of the skills-based intervention model has been seen at a number of levels. The theoretical principles explicit within cognitive behavioural interventions govern the structure, content and delivery of interventions. At the centre of such an approach was the notion that as certain *deficits* in affective, cognitive and interpersonal functioning are associated with offending, such deficits can, almost as a defining principle, be rectified. The type of clinical intervention best suited to addressing deficits was a structured, teaching approach which, whilst not denying the importance of a collaborative relationship with those delivering treatment, emphasised the importance of targeting deficits in thinking and behaviour through a skills-based approach. The deficits in appraisal or interpersonal functioning identified as intrinsically related to antisocial behaviour become the targets for intervention, addressed in more or less the same way as any other skill deficit is addressed. The focused and highly structured treatment which became widespread in the 1990s had as a core treatment principle the objective of teaching offenders to learn more adaptive thinking and behavioural styles.

Lipsey[22] in a meta-analytic review supported the notion that providing a treatment paradigm that offered a structured, cognitively and behaviourally orientated approach which also taught offenders concrete skills was likely to lead to reduced recidivism. Skills-based approaches, whilst being multi-modal in that they provided a range of treatment methods, all attempted to engage offenders through an overarching model. These included role play, pro-social modelling, cognitive rehearsal, the generation of cognitive and behavioural alternatives and the development of choice in the direction of favouring pro-social over antisocial alternatives.

Structure, consistency and treatment integrity

An important aspect of treatment development was the notion that unless the principles of effective programme design and delivery were adhered to, potentially serious ramifications could emerge. If drift occurred either in terms of the risk, need and responsivity criteria not being met or the content of the treatment being altered or adapted, the quality of interventions would be compromised and, significantly, their effectiveness reduced.[23,24] The result was the development of a system of highly structured, managed and monitored interventions. Within these interventions content was standardised to be delivered in largely identical, manualised programmes which contained an established number of sessions, each with its own specified delivery plan and treatment objectives. Whilst programmes vary in the extent to which every aspect of delivery is prescribed, they have at very least a structured format, clearly identified objectives and a specified plan for the delivery of each session. This format includes standard exercises and homework assignments, with a revision of learning points and session aims occurring at the end of each session and referred to at the start of the next.

Targets for change; what to treat

Maladaptive belief systems, cognitive biases and interpersonal skill deficits are regarded as a product of impoverished learning opportunities which do not represent underlying, immutable personality characteristics.[7,25] This concept has clear implications for what constitutes appropriate targets for treatment. An important piece of research by Dodge and Frame[26] indicated that the key cognitive process which differentiated aggressive from non-aggressive boys was the tendency to perceive hostile intent in the actions of others. Of particular relevance to the treatment of antisocial behaviour was not the diagnosis of being antisocial or psychopathic but on the psychological processes which were closely linked to violence. Blackburn[25] argued that it was these cognitive and interpersonal processes which mediated, or provided the link, between personality disorder and violent behaviour. Therefore it was these factors that should form targets for intervention. More importantly, cognitive and interpersonal processes were amenable to intervention and were directly related to violence. Attempting to unravel ingrained personality structures which may have limited causal relevance to antisocial behaviour lacks clinical relevance when the reduction in recidivism is the objective of treatment.

The emphasis of the debate about what constitutes a target for intervention is less on whether personality structure *per se* can change (although this remains an important clinical question), but on what aspects of personality are of relevance to offending. The position adopted by theorists such as Costa and McCrae[27] is that personality structure remains more or less intact over lifetime functioning. The focus of interest for intervention is the behaviours and psychological processes which mediate between personality traits, anti-social and violent behaviour and which of those behavioural, attitudinal and cognitive processes may be amenable to change.

Whilst empirical evidence supports the notion that personality traits are stable over lifespan,[28] the ability for individuals to manage, regulate and control behaviour across different environment or social conditions has been demonstrated by clinicians from different therapeutic paradigms. For those interested in the reduction of both criminogenic risk as well as the alleviation of psychological and personal distress, the *manifestation* of behavioural traits in the form of skills, attitudes, interests, habits and roles becomes a relevant and legitimate focus of enquiry.

Programme scope

Programme intervention initially developed from two main perspectives. Following the work of Ross, Fabiano and Ewles,[29] treatment was focused on deficits in thinking, problem-solving and interpersonal skills. These deficits were addressed rather than focusing on the offending behaviour *per se*. These programmes were referred to as Cognitive Skills programmes and aimed at offenders assessed as having deficits in these areas and typically were seen as relevant to violent, sex and drug offenders. Cognitive Skills programmes were followed by offence specific treatment which addressed the additional risk factors and treatment needs relevant to certain offences, particularly sex offences and violent offences. Programmes which address emotional regulation and anger control have also been introduced, with principles of risk, need and responsivity determining the dosage and intensity of treatment received and whether multiple programme intervention will be of value.

Case study

One of the most established and widely implemented treatment programmes is the Reasoning & Rehabilitation Programme which has been implemented in a variety of settings in several countries including Canada, the United States, England and many other countries throughout Europe. The Reasoning & Rehabilitation Programme (R&R)[29] is a structured cognitive behavioural treatment programme, specifically focusing on thinking skills. It adopts the theoretical position that the thinking skills which are necessary for pro-social adaption have not been acquired as part of the usual socialisation process in childhood. The programme adopts a broadly based learning approach to understanding the onset and maintenance of criminality and has, as its central premise, the assumption that essential skills can be acquired or learned through focused and structured intervention during adolescence or adulthood.

The main treatment targets for the programme include interpersonal problem-solving skills, social perspective taking, critical reasoning, rigid thinking and impulse control. The R&R Programme is delivered in 38 two-hour sessions, using a variety of teaching techniques, including role play, modelling and problem-solving exercises. The programme includes problem solving and creative thinking exercises as well as sessions which aim to enhance consequential thinking skills and moral reasoning. The programme focuses on the meta-cognition of offenders, that is, to encourage participants to think about their thinking. Those involved in the delivery programme are regarded as tutors or trainers rather than therapists.

Background

Alan is a 35-year-old male who is serving a 10-year sentence for discharge of a weapon in his workplace. The brief circumstances of the offence were that he was suspended from work after becoming threatening to his manager when feeling that he was being unfairly criticised. He immediately returned home where he kept a shotgun and returned to work with the weapon. After threatening his manager he discharged the shotgun. Nobody was hurt during the incident. Alan had only been employed two weeks at the time of the offence, and reports that he experienced considerable problems in his relationship with his wife because of his heavy drinking and lack of interest and attention towards the family. He considered that the suspension was grossly unjust and believed he had been singled out because he was an easy target. He also reported that he experienced bouts of depression and that his drinking was a result of this.

Assessment

Alan had five previous convictions for offences including violence, possession of drugs and causing criminal damage. His offending history stems back to the age of 15 and he had served two previous custodial sentences. A risk assessment took into account a variety of historical factors related to his offending and his employment and social history, indicating that Alan was considered to be classified as medium/high risk of further reoffending. An assessment of his offence-related needs indicated that his problem-solving and decision-making skills reflected an impulsive and rather reckless approach, he had limited concept of how his behaviour impacted upon others, he was unable to effectively regulate his temper and his behaviour was frequently unpredictable. He was unable to sufficiently anticipate the consequences of his behaviour across a variety of settings and tended to externalise responsibility for his social, vocational and interpersonal difficulties onto those around him, particularly his wife and former employer. Alan was considered suitable for the R&R Programme in that his risk category was deemed appropriate to the level and style of intervention adopted by the programme and he was assessed as having needs in the majority of the areas targeted. He agreed to participate in the programme on the grounds that he wanted to avoid going back to prison. Alan failed to see that his behaviour was unreasonable, given the circumstances, although he acknowledged that his previous behaviour reflected a pattern which he was unable to break.

The first 10 sessions of the treatment focused on problem solving. These were broken down into problem recognition, the definition and conceptualisation of 'a problem statement', the generation of alternatives, consequential thinking and an exploration of the potential biases or errors which can be made when attempting to assess a situation, including being able to separate fact from opinion. Initially Alan found the process monotonous and considered that it was largely irrelevant to his needs, which he felt would be resolved if others would adopt a more reasonable stance in their behaviour towards him. However, he did recognise that he experienced a considerable number of difficulties, particularly in relationships with other people. In addition, he found sessions on recognising and anticipating problems useful. For example, he stated that previously he only realised he had a problem when he was in the middle of an argument or after he had been fired from his job. He reported that being able to identify the internal and external cues which suggested that a problem may be escalating enabled him to take action before matters got out of hand. He was also able to reflect on and identify what the issue was, instead of just experiencing a vague sense of being 'pissed off' or 'stressed out'. Alan was particularly motivated in the session on how it was possible to misread or misinterpret social cues. For example, in an exercise involving generating hypotheses about why his visitor had failed to show up for his weekly visit , he was able to develop a range of ideas beyond his initial belief that the 'screws' wouldn't let her in. He also acknowledged that non-verbal cues could have a variety of meanings and tutors noted that he became particularly involved when brainstorming possible reasons why his partner had appeared subdued during a recent phone call (he had initially put this down to her being pre-occupied due to her having an affair).

In a series of role plays, Alan first observed tutors and then participated himself in role-playing how he could respond to a situation where he was subject to criticism by his employer. The first stage involved reframing some of his appraisals and structuring the event in a less arousing and anger-provoking way, recognising that his understanding of the situation and his beliefs that he was been purposely criticised and humiliated may only reflect one possible take of the situation. He was also able to follow a series of social skills steps which enabled him to respond assertively and confidently to his employer whilst at the same time being able to appreciate the perspective held by the employer. He reported that in doing so he felt more in control of himself, less frustrated, and empowered by the ability to restructure the interpretation of events. He felt that he had been able to express his needs, whereas previously any sense of emotional discomfort was expressed in escalating tension, frustration and anger.

Alan also held particularly rigid beliefs about violence as a legitimate problem-solving tool. This became more of a problem in treatment because he continued to hold on to the notion that if somebody was 'disrespectful' then the only viable response was threats of or actual violence. Whilst Alan continued to believe that in certain situations violence was legitimate, he was able to consider that other responses were at least available to him and that they may be even more successful in enabling him to achieve his ends. Of note was his observation that he was more able to see his own role in the problems he encountered and recognise his pattern of externalising blame. Furthermore, he reported being less suspicious of others whose actions he had frequently appraised as hostile and provocative.

At the post-course review, Alan reported that he was more able to evaluate situations without thinking in extremes and gave an example of how he responded to being left off the wing football team without perceiving injustice or being 'stitched up'. He reported that on a recent home leave that he had used the time constructively by visiting his probation officer and an alcohol support agency. In addition, he felt less pressurised by his associates who were trying to encourage him to spend the few days celebrating. Again, Alan reported that he was able to weigh up the advice of his friends and make his own decision about the best way to structure his leave.

A psychometric test battery had been implemented pre and post course and again at the three-month follow-up stage. This indicated that he had developed social perspective-taking skills and had developed more adept social problem-solving skills. It also suggested a less impulsive approach towards decision making and that his thinking style reflected a less justifying and minimising attitude and a reduced sense of entitlement. It also indicated less inclination to blame his problems on others. A behaviour checklist completed by his Personal Officer also reflected changes in his behaviour where he was seen as less volatile and aggressive and less prone to be influenced by those around him. He also enjoyed better relationships with staff. Some evidence did suggest, however, that his belief systems about his use of violence remained intact. It was recommended that as he had additional unmet treatment needs in this area he should attend a longer and more intensive programme which addressed the attitudes, constructs and value systems of violent offenders.

Conclusion

The word 'programme' tends to stir up emotive responses within those who find a concept of programming people an affront to the primacy of the therapeutic relationship. This reaction would be understandable if indeed the aims and scope of programme interventions were to create a conditioned yet law-abiding client group, whose freedom has somehow become subjugated in the process. However, the aims of programmes are not in fact vastly different from those of more traditional psychotherapy, with themes of choice, insight, improved social functioning and an internalised locus of control among the areas of common ground. Although the conceptual base on which programmes were developed has come a long way since their inception in the late 1980s, with the incorporation of a more inclusive range of treatment targets and methods, the suspicion of their agenda remains from certain quarters.[30]

Programmes have been criticised from a number of perspectives. From a conceptual point of view, critics of programmes argue that an approach based on a notion of teaching skills and rectifying cognitive deficits is doomed to failure in that this addresses symptoms and not causes. The concept of what constitutes treatment remains an interesting point of debate, although the relevance of the skills acquisition approach is one which is acknowledged across most psychotherapeutic paradigms, including cognitive analytic, dialectic behaviour as well as cognitive behavioural therapy.

A further criticism of the programme approach is a more fundamental critique of the meta-analytic approach upon which the 'What Works' framework was based and the over-reliance on studies from North America and Canada.[31] Furthermore, whilst there is a widely cited body of research suggesting the effectiveness of programmes,[32] until recently, very little evidence has been available regarding the effectiveness of this approach with incarcerated British offenders. Recent research findings from programmes run in the UK suggest significant treatment effects[33,34] as well as less conclusive evidence.[35]

The programme approach to intervention has clearly helped to refocus clinical work within forensic practice. Recent innovations in the field demonstrate the ability of programmes to adapt and modify in the light of experience. The focus on developmental factors and treatment outcomes such as healthy sexual functioning and positive lifestyles in programmes for sex offenders illustrates a change towards a more inclusive range of targets. This is in the context of a broadly based cognitive behavioural approach incorporating schema focused and social learning approaches to treatment. It is important that these developments are maintained, whilst keeping a critical eye on practice and guarding against the temptation of assuming that a narrow range of interventions within a single orthodoxy will lead to long-term and enduring change. A variable as complex as criminal behaviour, which is maintained by a diverse spectrum of cognitive, attitudinal, social and interpersonal factors, requires an intervention structure which is highly conscious of the difficulties in achieving and maintaining change. The principles for effective intervention and the emerging evidence base establishes a paradigm for ongoing developments in offender treatment.

References

1 Martinson R (1974) What Works? Questions and answers about prison reform. *The Public Interest.* **10**: 22–54.
2 Lipsey M (1995) What do we learn from 400 research studies on the effectiveness of treatment of juvenile delinquents? In: J McGuire (ed.) *What Works: reducing reoffending.* Wiley, London.
3 Losel F (1995) The efficacy of correctional treatment: a review and synthesis of meta evaluations. In: J McGuire (ed.) *What Works: reducing reoffending.* Wiley, London.
4 Blackburn R (1980) *Still Not Working? A look at recent outcomes in offending rehabilitation.* Paper presented at the Scottish Branch of the British Psychological Society's Conference on 'Deviance', University of Stirling, UK.
5 McGuire J and Priestley P (1985) *Offending Behaviour: skills and strategies for going straight.* Batsford, London.
6 Gendreau P and Ross RR (1985) Revivification of rehabilitation: evidence from the 1980s. *Justice Quarterly.* **4**: 349–407.
7 Andrews DA and Bonta J (1994) *The Psychology of Criminal Conduct.* Anderson, Cincinnati, OH.
8 Andrews DA (1989) Recidivism is predictable and can be influenced: using risk assessments to reduce recidivism. *Forum on Corrections Research.* **1**(20): 11–18.
9 Cooke DJ and Philip L (2001) To treat or not to treat? An empirical perspective. In: C Hollin (ed.) *Handbook of Offender Assessment and Treatment.* John Wiley & Sons, Chichester.
10 Andrews D (1995) Criminal conduct and effective treatment. In: J McGuire (ed.) *What Works: reducing reoffending.* Wiley, London.
11 Rice ME, Harris GT and Cormier CA (1992) An evaluation of a maximum security therapeutic community for psychopaths and other mentally disordered offenders. *Law and Human Behaviour.* **16**: 399–412.

12 Losel F (1993) The effectiveness of treatment in institutional and community settings. *Criminal Behaviour and Mental Health.* **3**(4): 416–37.

13 Andrews DA, Zinger I, Hoge RR *et al.* (1990) Does correctional treatment work? A clinically relevant and psychologically informed analysis. *Criminology.* **28**: 369–404.

14 McGuire J and Priestly P (1995) Reviewing 'What Works': past, present, and future. In: J McGuire (ed.) *What Works: reducing reoffending.* Wiley, London.

15 Blackburn R (1993) *The Psychology of Criminal Conduct.* Wiley, Chichester.

16 Bandura A (1977) *Social Learning Theory.* Prentice Hall, Englewood Cliffs, NJ.

17 Glueck S and Glueck ET (1950) *Unravelling Juvenile Delinquency.* Harvard University Press, Cambridge, MA.

18 Izzo RL and Ross RR (1990) Meta-analysis of rehabilitation programs for juvenile delinquents: a brief report. *Criminal Justice and Behaviour.* **17**: 134–42.

19 Garrett JC (1985) Effects of residential treatment on adjudicated delinquents. A meta-analysis. *Journal of Research in Crime and Delinquency.* **22**: 287–308.

20 Beck A, Rush AJ, Shaw BF *et al.* (1979) *Cognitive Therapy of Depression.* Guilford Press, New York.

21 Beck A (1999) *Prisoner of Hate: the cognitive basis of anger, hostility and violence.* HarperCollins, New York.

22 Lipsey MW (1992) The effect of treatment on juvenile delinquents: results from meta-analysis. In: F Losel, T Bliesener and D Bender (eds) *Psychology and Law: international perspectives.* de Gruyter, Berlin.

23 Grensheimer LK, Mayer JP, Gottschalk R *et al.* (1986) Diverting youths from the juvenile justice system: a meta-analysis of intervention efficacy. In: SJ Apter and A Goldstein (eds) *Youth Violence: programs and prospects.* Pergamon Press, Elmsford, NY.

24 Lipsey M (1995) What do we learn from 400 research studies on the effectiveness of treatment of juvenile delinquents? In: J McGuire (ed.) *What Works: reducing reoffending.* Wiley, London.

25 Blackburn R (1998) Psychopathy and the contribution of personality to violence. In: T Millon, R Simonsen, M Birket-Smith and RD Davis (eds) *Psychopathy: antisocial, criminal and violent behaviour.* Guilford Press, New York.

26 Dodge KA and Frame CL (1982) Social cognitive biases and deficits in aggressive boys. *Child Development.* **53**: 620–35.

27 Costa PT and McCrae RR (1994) Set in plaster? Evidence for the stability of adult personality. In: TF Heatherton and JL Weinberger (eds) *Can Personality Change?* American Psychological Association, Washington, DC.

28 Costa PT and McCrae RR (1988) Personality in adulthood: a six-year longitudinal study of self reports and spouse ratings on the NEO Personality Inventory. *Journal of Personality and Social Psychology.* **54**: 853–63.

29 Ross RR, Fabiano EA and Ewles CD (1988) Reasoning and rehabilitation. *International Journal of Offender Therapy and Comparative Criminology*. **32**: 29–36.

30 Fraser D (2002) Doubts about 'What Works': A Crime & Society Research Association (CSRA) Briefing Document. *Justice of the Peace*. **166**: 348–50.

31 Gorman K (2001) Cognitive behaviouralism and the holy grail: the quest for a universal means of managing offender risk. *Probation Journal*. **48**(1): 3–9.

32 Robinson D (1995) *The Impact of Cognitive Skills Training on Post-release Recidivism among Canadian Federal Offenders*. Correctional Services Canada, Ottawa.

33 Friendship C, Blud L, Erikson M *et al.* (2003) Cognitive-behavioural treatment for imprisoned offenders: an evaluation of HM Prison Service's cognitive skills programmes. *Legal and Criminological Psychology*. **8**: 103–14.

34 Friendship C, Mann R and Beech A (2003) The prison-based Sex Offender Treatment Programme – an evaluation. *Findings*. **205**. HM Prison Service Research, Development and Statistics Directorate.

35 Falshaw L, Friendship C, Travers R and Nugent F (2003) Searching for 'What Works': an evaluation of cognitive skills programmes. *Findings*. **206**. HM Prison Service Research, Development and Statistics Directorate.

Part Two

Mainly practice

Chapter 6

Thinking under fire: the prison therapeutic community as container

Andrew Downie

Introduction

The main pioneer of group analysis was SH Foulkes, and he developed much of his thinking about groups in a therapeutic community setting, Northfield hospital, which treated so-called shell-shocked soldiers during the Second World War. He succeeded Wilfred Bion at that establishment. Although the two developed their ideas about groups seemingly independently, these ideas finding an outlet in two distinct institutions (in Foulkes's case the Institute of Group Analysis, in Bion's the Tavistock Clinic), recently there has been an increasing rapprochement. For example, the group analyst Malcolm Pines[1] has co-edited two volumes looking at Bion's contribution to a psychodynamic understanding of what happens in groups. Colin James[2] added Winnicott's notion of holding to his comparison of Bion's thoughts on containment with Foulkes's concept of the matrix.

I share that interest, in particular Bion's idea about thinking. In the field of rehabilitation at present, there is a great deal of emphasis on interventions designed to help offenders change the way they think, or do not think. Outside of establishments such as Grendon, most of those interventions are based on cognitive behavioural principles. I seek to argue that there continues to be a need for the application of a psychodynamic understanding of thinking, and that the therapeutic community setting enables that application to be made.

It was Freud[3] who said that in order to avoid conscious awareness of conflict, some individuals avoid contact with difficult feelings through unthinking action. One of the men on B Wing, Ben, was serving life for killing three people. As a young man, seeking a new form of relationship as a reaction against a traumatic family background characterised by sudden and dramatic bereavements (for instance, he saw his sister kill herself by taking poison at the family meal table), he developed an obsessive attachment to a girlfriend. Believing that she was being unfaithful with his best friend, he went to this young man's house, stabbed him to death, and killed his two young housemates who came to investigate the disturbance.

Prior to these murders, the inmate, realising the mental torment he was going through, had made an appointment to see a psychiatrist, an appointment he did not keep. In therapy he talked about how he could not bear talking about his feelings: the terrible and tragic action that he took seemed to him at the time the only way out of his dilemma. To echo the title of this chapter, he could not contemplate thinking under fire.

Freud may well have highlighted the problem, but his ideas as to possible solutions, and those of others who have sought to work with offenders from a psychoanalytic or broader psychodynamic perspective, have taken a drubbing in recent years. 'What Works'[4] was an attempt to demonstrate which psychological interventions were successful in reducing reoffending. Its findings were not particularly encouraging for psychodynamic practitioners. It declared that there was no evidence that psychoanalysis or any of its derivatives worked, in terms of reducing reoffending. Instead, training programmes for offenders, delivered by tutors from an accompanying manual, based on ideas derived from cognitive behaviour therapy, became the order of the day. Several programmes have been developed for use in the Prison Service setting.

One of the most successful of these is the Sex Offender Treatment Programme.[5] It works on the premise that was presented at the start of this dissertation: that those who offend have problems with their thinking. It expands this idea in terms of individuals' core beliefs; how people see themselves and others.

> 'For each core belief, people will have a number of intermediate beliefs. These are referred to in our model as schema. A schema is a category of related attitudes, assumptions and rules. The precise nature and content of someone's schemas will come from their core beliefs and life experiences.'

There is congruence here with analytic thinking; hardly surprising since one of CBT's prime advocates is Aaron Beck, who trained as an analyst. What is different is the core belief that participants can learn about their schema, and how to modify them, didactically, rather than evocatively, as would hopefully happen in 'free-floating' therapy. I would not wish to suggest that all learning has to be experiential, and that nothing taught has any place; indeed, the style of teaching called for by such programmes, using Socratic questioning, encouraging group participation, is potentially sympathetic or complementary to group analytic methods. Rawlinson[6] describes how such programmes have been integrated into a non-residential therapeutic community with a strong group analytic bias.

I would argue, though, that in terms of helping offender patients develop their thinking, there continues to be a place for psychodynamic interventions, where the knowledge that comes through new thoughts is arrived at evocatively, that is, through the exchanges that are part of therapeutic relationships, especially in the context of a therapeutic community. I am relieved that we seem to have moved away from the simplistic acceptance of 'What Works' to an acceptance that Grendon works too. This is demonstrated by the opening of a second therapeutic community establishment, HMP Dovegate.

I would further argue that knowledge gained evocatively has a certain distinct advantage. Because it is knowledge gained through the process of relating to another or others in therapy, a process involving concepts such as transference, projection, and projective identification, it enables the thinker to develop the skill of thinking about what is happening for him in relation to others, particularly in anxiety-provoking situations, whilst it is happening. The analyst Wilfred Bion,[7] himself a pioneer therapeutic community practitioner, referring aptly to working with shell-shocked soldiers, called this thinking under fire.

In support of my argument, I describe the key contribution made by Bion to a psychodynamic understanding of thinking, the relevance of his ideas to work with offender patients, and then how a therapeutic community can provide the matrix to enable thinking to develop.

Bion's theory of thinking

The Symingtons[8] describe Bion's principal concern as the application of thought to emotional experience which happens for us all in the context of relationships, the kind of experience that inmate Ben, mentioned earlier, found so difficult, certainly whilst it was happening to him. He could not think under fire. The Symingtons say:

> 'So the catalyst which gives rise to the emotional experience is the link between one human being and another. It is out of this emotional experience that either a thought process or a discharge will take place.'

In Ben's case, the three murders were a discharge.

Bion's emphasis on the thinking process in therapy seems to have been driven by a desire to arrive at the truth. He believed that the truth, when faced, and as an object relations thinker, faced with others, as in an individual or group therapeutic situation, would lead to mental growth. In biblical terms, the truth shall set you free. This is relevant to men at Grendon. In their criminal activities they may have sought to evade detection, or not told the truth about themselves. Armed robbery, for example, is frequently an act of deception, where the robber will convince his victim that he will use the weapon when in fact he would not. If the weapon were a frozen cucumber in a carrier bag, as in the case of one former resident, then it would not be much use as a weapon anyway. But the truth is usually deeper than that. The offence rarely, if ever, says the truth, the whole truth and nothing but the truth about the man. Often it is the means to enable him to present a 'false self' to the world.

For Bion, finding out and accepting the truth meant moving from avoiding pain to an acceptance of suffering. He described this as an oscillating process between what Melanie Klein described as the paranoid-schizoid and depressive positions. Men's offences often represent attempts to avoid pain and project it into their victims, and the oscillations between this position and one of facing pain and suffering are evident in the cycles that the work goes through. There will be a time when there will be a lot of work on difficult material being carried out on small groups, there will be lots of dialogue on wing meetings, people will be being challenged for bad behaviour, and supported through particular difficulties, and then something will happen: maybe a member of staff will go off sick, or residents might feel that we or the prison in general is being unfair to them in some way, and there will be a retreat from the advances that have been made. There will be rumours that there are drugs on the wing. Discussion about the issue will be difficult. Nobody (at least not at first) will want to 'grass' on anybody, indicating that we have gone back to default prison mode. People might talk about others being compromised, unable to talk for fear of what somebody else knows about them. Staff will also go back to default prison mode, and speculate about possible guilty parties. Residents will insist, 'Staff must know what's going on. Just do something, will you?' If we as a staff group manage to refrain from precipitate action, sooner or later some new thinking will emerge out of the frustration. The cycle begins again.

Bion used symbols to represent individuals' patterns of relatedness to one another, L being love, H hate and K the knowing function. Coming from the object relations school, he believed that we are all essentially relationship-seeking, and that the exchanges between us can be described in these terms. He added K, the thinking function, because he believed we wanted to know about ourselves and others, and the links between us. If an inmate has been caught for, or confessed to, using drugs, in his account to the wing, he will often say he did it just to get 'out of it', an indication that the levels of L, H and K were getting too much, and he wanted to attack the K, or linking, function. Drugs on the wing usually represent a minus-K situation. 'Getting out of it' on drugs could be seen as a way of avoiding thinking and attacking linking.

When we are making links with others, then we are both having an emotional experience and developing thinking. When we resist that process, then we have –K.

In my experience, –K situations come about when community members do not feel sufficiently contained; for example, when we have staffing difficulties, or when changes are afoot in the prison regime, and anxieties heighten about Grendon losing its special therapeutic status. Bion thought that the concept of containment was vital in the development of thinking. Following object relations principles, he moved away from the one-body psychology of Freud. Thinking is the result of at least two people's activity; they come together to produce a third: the thought itself. This process begins between mother and infant. The latter has innate predisposition to suck. This is defined as a preconception. The mother provides the breast: a realisation. The mating of the two produces a conception: the third. The child is beginning to develop a model of how his or her world works.

The infant will seek out the parent to respond to and contain other needs, primitive fears and anxieties, and angry feelings aroused by separation. Hopefully the parent will respond helpfully to expressions of distress. Further preconceptions will meet with realisation. In Bion's complicated quasi-mathematical language the child's beta elements, his or her raw, unprocessed sense impressions, will go through the mother's alpha function, her reverie, her attention to the child, and will be transformed there and given back in a form the child can manage. This is the process of projective identification in action. The child will begin to internalise an impression of the parent as responsive and caring, and will begin to develop his or own ability to contain difficult feelings. The contained gradually becomes the container.

This is a vital process if the next developmental stage is to be mastered: the ability to think. According to Bion, thoughts develop at the point of frustration, when a conception does not meet with a realisation, when there is no breast. In order not to experience overwhelming anxiety when the process of projective identification-reintrojection seems to have broken down, the child will need to think up the idea of a breast. This will depend on having had a good enough experience of the breast in the beginning. For Bion, however, the end aim of the process was not total independence of thinking in the individual: we are naturally relationship-seeking. We need an ongoing sense of being contained within relationships; then almost paradoxically we can learn how to tolerate frustration, pain and shame. The therapeutic setting provides such an opportunity for containment, but the principle of non-gratification provides an opportunity to experience frustration, and to learn to think under fire.

Bion was especially interested in psychotic thinking. His ideas need some translation for them to be helpful in the forensic setting. Gallwey[9] observes that when the early environment is not only inadequate, but when the child's attempts to project uncomfortable aspects of himself into the parent are met by retaliation, through physical, sexual or emotional abuse, or abandonment either literal or through psychological collapse:

> 'early projective identification fails both as a defence and as a link, and a particular type of malfunction develops which differs from both psychotic and neurotic equivalents . . . such an individual when able to do so starts treating the environment as if it were part of his psychic property, in order to achieve equilibrium and avoid fragmentation of the self into psychosis.'

This can lead, in Gallwey's view, to:

- enforced or subversive occupation of a substitute container and/or takeover of its contents
- triumph over a substitute container with cruel subjugation or violent annihilation.

A former community resident described how as a child he would run away from the care home where his mother had placed him. He would run home, but just hang around outside, peering through the windows. If he went in, experience told him that his mother would hand him over to the authorities. As an adolescent and adult, he became a prolific burglar. Another man is being assessed by staff. In the course of the meeting, he describes how much he wants to be like another man in the community, who he sees as having done well, but he feels is emotionally distant from him. 'I don't know how to break into him,' he says. He too is a burglar. The challenge in therapy therefore is for staff and residents to work together to create an environment that is sufficiently containing to hold on to men whilst they work on these issues.

The community as container

As a group analyst, I believe that each man will bring with him into the community his characteristic pattern of relating to the world, and will demonstrate this in his dealings with other residents and staff. As illustrated in particular by the second brief case example above, some of this pattern will parallel his offending. The community needs to contain his projective identifications, and feed them back to him so he can think about them – under fire.

Furthermore, I think that each individual's pattern of communication will combine together to make up what Foulkes[10] described as the matrix:

> 'The matrix is the hypothetical web of communication and relationship in a given group. It is the common shared ground which ultimately determines the meaning and significance of all events and upon which all communications and interpretations, verbal and non-verbal rest.'

It is known[11] that Foulkes chose the word matrix deliberately because of its derivation from the Latin mater, or mother. It is the matrix that acts as container.

The matrix can be described as building up at various levels: the 'here and now' of what is being said and done, the transferential level of how those exchanges might represent members' families of origin, the 'projective' level where people put bits of themselves into others ('why do you let him rent a space in your head?' is sometimes said to someone about an interpersonal conflict), and finally the level of Jung's collective unconscious, where the pattern of communication is similar to an ancient archetypal story. In a well-established community, such as B Wing in Grendon, there is the potential for great richness of experience for community members to draw upon.

If the matrix is strong enough, then it should be able to sustain those that make it up through difficult times, and continue to enable its members to reflect on their experiences through these difficult times: to help them continue to think under fire.

Clinical vignette: the community meeting – a sociodrama in three acts

Act one

The community room is large, rectangular, and has nearly 50 seats set around its edge, with an open space in the middle. It is uncarpeted. It is B Wing's proud boast (more of a projection than a reality, no doubt) that A Wing, our sister community across the corridor, may have a carpet, but its main function is to conceal issues that should be talked about, unlike B Wing, where we have open and honest communication.

The chairman, John, begins the meeting. Although we follow what is described as a Maxwell Jones democratic therapeutic community model, with residents occupying key positions such as wing chair, I seek to work from a group analytic perspective and part of my mental preparation is to remind myself that I should be there with him as the facilitator of the large group. It is a shared responsibility to create and preserve the therapeutic space.

The meeting has a business function, and that often represents a safe way for people to let go of the side, and skate out onto the ice. The education officer mentions some courses that are running, some certificates for achievement in sports activities are given out, and the community comments and votes on inmates who are applying for jobs. I read out the staff feedback on some residents' assessments. Participants in the complementary activities that the wing and Grendon in general offers (psychodrama, art therapy) describe what has been happening in their groups. This takes less than half an hour of our scheduled hour and a half: there is no more formal business. John then utters the fateful words, 'Wing open,' and the potential for chaos, for the psychotic anxieties associated with large groups, begins to rise.

Act two

There is a brief silence, punctuated by some coughing and shuffling. It looks like some people are getting ready to let go of the side. One of the feedbacks earlier had been about the inter-wing meeting, a forum to discuss issues of common concern between staff and inmates across the prison. The B Wing representative has said that the flow of information is all one way at the moment, it's all staff telling inmates how it will be, no real exchange of ideas, how Grendon is supposed to be.

His comments tap into a general mood of discontent. The subject of money that had been promised to the wing for new furniture and fittings, that has not yet arrived, is raised. 'Other wings have had it,' one man says. The image of B Wing as Beirut, i.e. the current prison trouble spot, is cited as the reason for our being out of favour. One of the communities has to be the scapegoat, the container for the others' projections: it happens to be our turn. The general mood of the wing seems to be flat: a kind of sullen, depressed anger. Who listens anyway?

Damian, a resident who has in the past expressed a wish for a nice normal environment with net curtains covering the bars on the windows, and a carpet for the meeting room, in the hope of a place where, as he says, 'people don't fart and burp all the time', asks me what I think about the situation: 'We're always going on about this, nobody seems to care and nothing gets done.' The spotlight is on me. 'Come on Andy, get it sorted,' another voice calls. What I really want to do is think, but I feel I am being pushed into action.

What thoughts I do have tell me that this conversation is not just about the standard of décor, it is also about therapeutic space. It is a reflection of conversations that have gone on at other levels about the staffing crisis, about our new governor's departure after just a few months in the job, and his farewell letter describing how he could not cope, about the resignations of the Director of Therapy, the Senior Probation Officer, and the psychologist on my wing that have followed. Will the place carry on?

I need to respond both concretely and symbolically, I think. This is not the time to be a blank screen, which isn't my style anyway. I say words to the effect that I can identify with people's struggles to go about things in the right way, as they have done over this money for improvements. I wonder aloud how many of them have tried to do the right thing in the past, but have felt ground down and gave in to the chaos. I say I will do what I can about the money, but at the end of the day my job is to be the wing therapist, and as the therapist I wonder what happens to people when they feel like this: ground down by forces more powerful than them. In the past of course they have acted through their offences as a way of demonstrating their power, and their need to avoid a stronger version of the psychic pain that is finding muted expression now.

I am lonely on the ice, and I am inviting others to join me. A few pairs of eyes go up to the ceiling at my response, but hands stay clasped to the side for a while. Damian says, 'But therapy still gets done.' I agree, but wonder if it's harder in present circumstances. Feedback from small groups recently has tended to emphasise the sullen, angry, depressed mood on the wing.

Act three

As if to prove my point, what seems like an uncomfortable silence follows. John invites comments from anybody else. An inmate, Mark, has been brooding about what he sees as a personal injustice. The prison officer who is his key worker has refused to endorse his application for a therapy bonus payment for being in therapy for over a year. She does not think that his attitude has been conducive to his progress in therapy. He thinks he is being 'dug out' because he had accused her of having a bitchy attitude to him. Some inmates agree with him, taking this as yet another example of the lack of care that seems to be available at the moment. Then an inmate close to release, facing his own struggles with outside agencies over what he sees as them trying to place unjust restrictions on him through conditions attached to his release on licence, says to him: 'Come on, Mark, it's not really the money.'

I begin to think that my question about what happens for people when they feel let down might have some relevance, and through Mark there might be an attempt at some answers. The community works some more with Mark and brings him to the point of acknowledging that one of his difficulties is how he thinks, feels and acts when he is 'right'. Mark's crime was to arrange the killing of his partner after he found out she had had a relationship with another man. He had several affairs, but in his mind she was not allowed to pay him back in kind. When he is right, in his mind, he is justified in attacking. It is not enough for him just to think he is right: in displays of narcissistic omnipotence, others have to experience Mark's rightness. Somebody says that all of this just hides how worthless Mark feels he is, but can't admit. Wanting a therapy bonus is just a cover-up. He struggles with being told 'no'. Mark looks thoughtful for a moment, and nods in agreement . . . John, the chairman, killed his wife, driven by obsessive jealousy over her 'preferring' their son to him, and he says ruefully that he can identify with what Mark is saying, and what is being said to him. I point out what I see as the link between what Mark was talking about and the earlier content of the meeting. People were saying they wanted better. It was with a sense of 'You lot should give us these things', but with no real sense that they deserved better. What hurt about the present deprivation was that it reminded people of their sense of worthlessness. Mark was not even worth a £10 therapy bonus. He has actually been heard to say that he deserved hanging.

The community has managed to turn some frustration into thinking, albeit painful thoughts. I am reminded that this thinking has been achieved at a price. Shortly before the meeting ends, Paul says angrily that sometimes he thinks that staff see therapy as a way of turning him and others into 'soft cunts'. 'We'll just talk about things and not kick off.' He gives voice to the fear that maybe it is all about being more ready to feel pain. He has agreed with chairman John, who has said, 'I never want to be hurt again.'

Why does Grendon 'work' (not, of course, that it does all the time or for everybody)? Foulkes's first law of group dynamics still seems to apply, that collectively the members of the community form the norm from which individually they deviate. Bion and other therapeutic community pioneers found that expecting their patients not to be just patients but co-therapists as well – containing others as well as being contained – proved to be a powerful factor in their recovery. After all, they are the experts in their own condition.

Staff, however, should receive the credit they deserve. Billow,[12] a group therapist heavily influenced by Bion, said:

> 'Ultimately what holds the group together is the therapist's ever expanding understanding of the psychic reality of the group and its members, and the therapeutic success in interesting others in reaching and deepening such understanding, however painful and unwelcome.'

The ability of the staff teams at Grendon to receive the projections on to them, to hold these and think about them, and to present them back in a modified form that can be processed, and can indicate they understand, rather than condemn, the community resident, acts as a powerful model of thinking under fire.

Concluding comments

Many men, after a few weeks, especially after they have moved on to one of the larger wings after their stay on the induction and assessment unit, begin to express their disappointment in Grendon. It's not what they hoped for; staff are just like those in mainstream prisons. Their preconceptions have not been met with a realisation. It is important then not to meet their attempts at rejection with retaliation, but for staff and inmates to seek to contain their projections, then the process of helping them to think about their frustrations while they are experiencing them, the process Bion called 'thinking under fire', can begin.

Community members' preconceptions can then lead to new realisations, and the risk can be taken collectively to think new thoughts. Shortly before he left the community, making a progressive move to a lower security category prison, Ben had to hand out his beloved caged bird, as the new establishment did not allow them. Ben cried; and what is more, he told others he had done so. 'I never thought I would have told people that,' he said.

References

1 Lipgar RM and Pines M (eds) (2003) *Building on Bion: branches.* Jessica Kingsley, London.
2 James DC (1994) Holding and containing in the group society. In: D Brown and L Zinkin (eds) *The Psyche and the Social World: developments in group analytic theory.* Routledge, London.
3 Freud S (1914) *Remembering, Repeating and Working Through.* Standard Edition of the Complete Works of Sigmund Freud, Vol. 12. Hogarth Press, London.
4 McGuire J (ed.) (1995) *What Works: reducing reoffending.* Wiley, London.
5 HM Prison Service Offending Behaviour Programmes Unit (1998) *Sex Offender Treatment Programme: treatment manual.* HM Prison Service, London.
6 Rawlinson D (1999) Group analytic ideas: extending the group matrix into TCs. In: P Campling and R Haigh (eds) *Therapeutic Communities: Past, Present and Future.* Jessica Kingsley, London.
7 Young R (1997) *Group Relations: an introduction* (Internet book). Available at www.human-nature.com/myyoung/papers/paper99.html
8 Symington J and Symington N (1996) *The Clinical Thinking of Wilfred Bion.* Routledge, London.
9 Gallwey P (1991) Social maladjustment. In: J Holmes (ed.) *Textbook of Psychotherapy in Psychiatric Practice.* Churchill Livingstone, Edinburgh.
10 Foulkes S (1964) *Therapeutic Group Analysis.* Allen & Unwin, London.
11 Powell A (1994) Towards a unifying concept of the group matrix. In: D Brown and L Zinkin (eds) *The Psyche and the Social World: developments in group analytic theory.* Routledge, London.
12 Billow R (2003) *Relational Group Psychotherapy.* Jessica Kingsley, London.

Chapter 7

Working with the unbearable

Liz McLure

Abstract

Anything that can be thought about has already been done. By extension, all of our most awful fantasies have already been enacted. How is it possible to bear the knowledge of having done some of these things and how is it possible to work with those who have done them? This chapter looks at the complex and powerful feelings that are aroused in work with male offenders and considers the importance of acknowledging both the conscious responses and the unconscious transference and countertransference.

Introduction

The work takes place in a therapeutic community prison. The group is one of five in the wing. Each small group meets at the same time three times a week. These groups are interspersed with short wing feedback meetings and a longer large group experience twice a week. The continuity of staff assigned to each group and the structure and frame of the community provides the social milieu that enables therapy to take place. The groups are places where the dilemmas of working and living together are explored; the dynamic tension is palpable and at times explosive. Re-enactments of traumatic situations in the lives of the men are played out continuously in the here and now of relationships on the wing and in the prison as a whole. When the status quo is upset and the collective vulnerability is exposed, the cohesion is lost and the community easily regresses to a position of fight/flight, with scapegoating, pairing, splitting, intense projective identification, and a push against the rules and those who hold or represent the power. The small groups attempt to provide a safer and more personal place for further exploration and analysis of these happenings and the relationship to the internal world of each individual. The search for understanding and meaning is both exciting and threatening. It is often chaotic, yet despite this we continue to come together at the allotted time to sit in a circle on low soft blue chairs placed on a square 'island' of incongruous red and yellow patterned carpet in the middle of the large community room. Therapy is taken very seriously. The setting may be surreal for group therapy, but the stories and experiences of working here are very real.

The external world intrudes to give a flavour of reality about how these men are viewed; their shame and society's shame resonates in every group. 'We are the people who have done these nasty horrible deeds and inflicted great pain and suffering on our fellow human beings. We have been tried and convicted of this, we cannot hide our actions under any banner that would legitimise what we did,' commented one of the men in the group.

The prison offers the containment required for this group to undertake therapy. There is a need for the extra safety that this external boundary provides; they had no boundaries in the past and frequently violated the boundaries of others. Their past destructive and deviant coping strategies when distressed or bored are what led them to being here. They got what they wanted, but were never satisfied. Many admit that they would not have stopped offending if they had not been caught. They are all familiar with offending behaviour as a means of survival. Exploring a different way to survive without violating others is new and threatening. It is all they know. Acting out in unsociable ways continues until better ways are found to be. What becomes apparent all too soon is that the most difficult thing to talk about, the most unbearable part of the therapy, is the past – how did they get to be like this, what set them off on this path? They realise the need to re-experience the emotions and feelings contained in memories of the past that have been defended against at all costs. Defended against, but habitual and symbolised in their offences. These men were halted or derailed from the normal course of psychological development at critical stages in their lives and did not learn how to contain feelings of hurt, pain, rage, despair and hatred from the past. They were often deprived of love, care, empathic understanding, nurture and stability in their lives. They were troubled and got into trouble. They were terrified and learned how to terrorise. They were shamed and humiliated and they learned how to denigrate others. They faced physical death and annihilation of the psyche and they killed and tortured. They identified with their aggressors in order to survive. 'No one gave a f**k about me, why should I give a f**k about them.'

They take time to settle and to realise that the macho image of the survivor is no longer required. This comes with the development of trust and safety in the small groups. The 'strong and brave' man here is one who will talk and cry if need be. They will not ridicule each other, as they know that they need to do the same. There is respect for those who are serious about therapy and who wish to explore their darker side and to expose their vulnerable core to learn how to bear their emotional pain. Through the group they see themselves relative to others and appreciate the change which comes from being able to integrate and tolerate each other and as a result all aspects of the self.

To illustrate the complexity of this work I have included examples based on material from over 500 group sessions. No names are used and some details changed to maintain anonymity and confidentiality. Those who could be more easily identified, i.e. in vignettes, have given consent to the use of their stories for this purpose. I have also included some of my own transference/counter-transference reactions to the group. The group often works at a very primitive level; some of the deeper and more painful aspects of their communications in the group usually emerge in my dreams. Often I will find myself having a recurring dream about someone in the group prior to a disclosure or major piece of work from that individual. The dream is usually in context as the content has been lurking around in the matrix for some time and just waiting to be owned and voiced by one of the men. Sometimes my dreams are sexual, sometimes they are full of violence, mostly they are frightening and at times very disturbing. I have learned to trust and make use of these dreams in supervision as an aid to understanding the group projections and transferences to me and what that means in terms of other object relations in their lives. This is particularly useful for those who have got tangled up in their libidinal and aggressive drives or where the libidinal aspects are split off and displaced completely into their other offences, e.g. arson. This is a vital part of the therapy for them and for me and can make sense of what is going on in the group. Communications of this nature may be returned to the group, not as presented here but in a more digested, processed form – in interpretations when appropriate or, if pertinent to an individual, written in their six-monthly assessment. This is a disclosure of my countertransference as opposed to a factual disclosure, in that it is interpersonal and specific to the relationship with them.

> 'Thoughtful countertransference disclosure is a useful tool in psychotherapy with adult survivors of childhood sexual (and other) abuse. Because these clients come to any new relationship with assumptions based on their experiences in earlier exploitative, abusive and non mutual relationships, the use of the new therapeutic relationship to undo old patterns and create new ways of relating is a critical component of the psychotherapy.'[1]

The core trauma – take two boys and give them a life of hell

Can you imagine what it is like to be beaten and neglected by your mother, to have your bones broken, to be left hungry and dirty in your cot screaming – fighting for survival and not yet two years old? You are rescued by being put into care. You experience further beatings, emotional neglect and punishment, but you are fed and the care given is consistent if not necessarily good. You then suffer a traumatic separation from your newfound carer, she lies to you, and abandons you to a series of foster-carers. You are now four years old and struggling to make sense of your experiences. Your behaviour is troublesome, you are misunderstood and punished further and more frequently. The adults responsible for your care do not break the cycle of abuse, they continue it. The 'siblings' you share with tease and taunt you, you are on your own, if you are to survive you have to adapt and you learn to be self-reliant. You trust no one. You learn to lie, to cheat, to steal. You get what you want, you learn how to give yourself pleasure and comfort in this way. Life, of course, does not get easier, you suffer further traumatic near-death experiences. The terror from earlier fear of annihilation shoots up into your psyche again and again. Glue, drugs, alcohol and dangerous pursuits keep you going. You have lots of casual relationships, you pump out your frustrations during sex, intimacy is never achieved. You are 'rescued again' by someone who cares about you and wants a relationship. You struggle to share yourself with any other completely – why should you trust? You believe you are unlovable. You cannot commit fully to the relationship. Intimacy is intolerable, you could get hurt. Distance is intolerable to your partner, she rejects you. Devastation! What do you do with these feelings of being abandoned, alone, terrified, humiliated, isolated, lost, and unlovable? You are still relatively young, only 24. You are lost and you lose it, the rage and hurt of the tiny child within explodes in a powerful, destructive, uncontained way. You rob and kick a man to death. He is drunk, defenceless, weak and vulnerable, his life had no meaning and no value – just like yours.

Can you imagine being brought up in a house where your mother is beaten and discarded by your father? You, too, suffer terrible beatings. Anything that is loved is destroyed. Your mother is depressed and unable to resist or protect either herself or you. You hate her for her vulnerability and her inadequacy. She takes her temper out on you. You blame her for your father not loving you both; he is not there to bear the brunt of your feelings for him. You get a new stepdad. He blackmails your mother into having sex by threatening you. You hate him and you hate your mother for all of this, the bit of you that loved her and needs her is put in a box for safekeeping. New siblings get a better deal, they are loved and special. Your envy and hatred of them is added to your rage and resentment towards mother. You put that in another box. Your only consistent and safe relative dies – loving someone ends in disaster, this is painful. You put that in another box, one that is already full to overflowing. Feelings are dangerous and destructive, getting close to another is threatening. Sexual feelings become confusing and distress you. How can you be attracted to and have positive feelings towards the thing that is the source of your pain and you hate the most (women)? You hate your own feelings. You feel inadequate. You are lost and seek absolution and a wish for great power. You get preoccupied with death and evil. You torture and kill your pets. You mutilate your own body in a ritualistic way. You are the most dangerous man you know. You want revenge and you welcome death. Your hatred leads you to attack the things that your mother loves and are symbolic of her sex and your feelings of inadequacy and being like her. You beat, torture and rape her daughter, your envied and hated sister, you are all-powerful and you get revenge for the rape and pillage of your psyche. You try to kill yourself but your suicide attempt is thwarted as you are found – but not yet saved.

These two brief vignettes give an account of the typical life stories and an indication of the complex psychopathology and personality organisation of the men in the group. Each comes into focus and emerges from time to time against the backdrop of the group. Add another six equally disastrous life accounts and you have a typical group. The stories take time to unfold and the connections between the past, the offence and current ways of relating are pieced together gradually. The symbolic nature of the offence is often clearer to the observers in the group; allowing the individual to recognise, own and understand their own offending behaviour takes patience and time. It is a slow and painful process. This is not your 'typical group analytic' group and requires something different of the conductor in response to the way the group explores 'issues'.

> 'In 1980 Kernberg proposed that whereas individual treatment tends to activate "higher level" object relations involving transference neuroses, group interaction probably elicits aggressive and sexual fantasies on a primitive regressed level. The group also offers a treatment modality which provides support, encouragement and reality-orientated feedback which can be conducive to growth by creating a safe atmosphere in which to explore and harness the potentially violent eruptions.'[2]

The early days – when I first participated in the life of the group

When I started work with this group over four years ago, they related to each other in a very abusive way. Everything that could not be contained was projected out and acted into on the group. They would humiliate and shame each other, abuse verbally and emotionally, threaten with physical violence, bully, punish by exclusion, groom (seduce) and manipulate, lie, deceive and steal. There was a pecking order too: armed robbers were at the top, the 'most respected' in the system list, then came the murderers, the rapists, the paedophiles and at the bottom of the list the child killers. In the system, as in society, the lives of those at the bottom of the list were made hell. This group was no exception; no one wanted to be seen as the lowest of the low or to be seen as similar in any way to those perceived to be the lowest. All aspects of self which could identify with these offences were denied and projected onto those who conveniently had the label to be hated. Few talked of the violations they had committed and got away with. They were a destructive, abusive group. There was little space for reflection, no empathy or warmth towards each other, no concern or understanding of why they did what they did and why they were the way they were. They were both victims and perpetrators, desperately struggling not to be anyone else's victim by being a perpetrator. All without lasting relief from the constant projection and re-introjection of the bad, nasty, cruel, sadistic, vengeful aspects of their rage and pain.

It was my task to halt the cycle of abuse in our relationships with the group and each other. I could not afford to collude with or rise to the bait with an attacking defence on my part. It was a constant struggle to maintain my integrity and contain and control my own feelings of rage, disgust, despair, mistrust, fear and anxiety. Modelling care, compassion, respect, genuine interest, empathic concern, listening and being heard was hard work. This was doubly difficult as most of these men were betrayed as boys,[3] have experienced abuse in 'the system' or care institutions and have no trust in any person who symbolises authority. Most had poor or non-existent relationships with their mothers and were rejected by women throughout their lives. My gender was against me too. At times I acted into the abusive role; I am only human and not perfect. I acknowledged my mistakes to the group, fostering a culture of openness and honesty. To deny my misdemeanours would have served to widen the trust gap and leave them with a denial on my part. 'The mother who can take in her infant's state of mind, attend to, sustain and think about it, who can understand and know her child and respond appropriately may be introjected as someone who can tolerate pain, imbue it with meaning and thereby modify the experience of experience (sic).'[4]

The secure 'play pen' and the therapeutic space had to be created and maintained to enable a degree of trust, one of the hardest things for these men to achieve. Most want this yet fear it; they want intimacy with another but are terrified of abuse and rejection. They long for safety and warmth, care and understanding, but often do not know what to do with it. They wallow in the attention they receive from the conductor in the group. They vie for this 'special' place, yet resist any one-to-one connection in the group. The competition is rife at times, especially following breaks. My attention is torn every which way; I am fought over like a coveted toy. Keeping them in check without inflicting narcissistic wounds is a tricky business. I felt like the 'old woman who lived in a shoe' having so many children and not knowing what to do. This left me at times feeling paralysed, neglectful, depressed, and so conflicted that it was impossible to think and hold myself together as well as the group. They needed firm containment, and being kept in check demanded greater emotional resilience and strength from me, tested continuously. It is a frightening thing to challenge those who step out of line, yet to not do it instils fear and despair in the group. Whilst they were taking off their 'macho' overcoats I had to work towards dispelling the myth of the projected stereotypical imago of me as a 'white, middle class, lesbian, man-hater, do-gooder with a degree in something'. They tested me and tried to show me up in the larger community. They wanted to humiliate and denigrate me in public just to see how I would react. It was OK for them to do this to me, but if any others were critical of me they defended me to the hilt. The struggles with dependency and intimacy had begun. I knew that I was to be both loved and hated with a passion.

On my first group I was told by one man, 'Don't talk psychobollocks!' This was in part to put me in my place, to disempower me, but it also served the purpose of teaching me how to relate to them in a way that would be meaningful. I knew that if I survived the first group intact and did not run scared or become defensive straight off that I could be accepted by this group. For them there was safety in numbers and they could easily exclude me if they wanted to. I took his advice and found ways to use their words and behaviour in the metaphors used to describe the process of what was happening in the group, particularly the hostile attacks on the group, the therapy and me. I would use phrases like 'holding the group hostage with words', 'stabbing us in the head', 'lobbing in a few grenades and watching the sparks fly', 'getting me to drop my boundaries' (seduce) and (for telling me secrets of the group) 'dealing sweets on the group'. The group would play with these and developed some useful metaphors and analogies of their own. 'Would you trust a wolf in a field of sheep just because it told you it had turned vegetarian?' – a phrase used by one man when asking another to consider his risk factors.

Subtlety and metaphor does not always work, particularly with the more concrete thinkers, and a direct approach is needed to get a point across. This takes courage as I have to face my fear of the reaction to say what needs to be said. Normally a group would challenge those who step out of line. However, here they often 'compromise' each other by holding secrets regarding minor misdemeanours and rule breaking or they fear a sneak attack or revenge taking in the way it happens in the system. Violence is a real threat here. Some fear 'bringing it on' in the group as they would lose their place if they 'lost it' and hit someone. Thus the pull to collude with others is immense. They fear and respect their own and each other's vulnerability and dangerousness.

Challenging their behaviour is like outing an abuser; it feels abusive and you then sit in their shoes for a while, having identified with them in your exposure of them. You also identified with their victim and reacted to what was put into you. The cycle of abuse can be understood. You begin to understand the principles and the motivation for revenge to get rid of the shame, rage, guilt and humiliation. You carry something for them now, it was perhaps not yours to carry in the first place, you are seen as the one who has wronged, but it is your burden until it can be understood and re-interpreted back into the group.

Holding offensive (to us) knowledge about others and what they have done challenges our internal boundaries to the limit. Unable to hold this much pain, terror, denigration, humiliation, shame, disgust and despair, sometimes we leak as a result and identify with the aggressor and project this onto ourselves as the muted self object of the aggressor(s) or onto others, an object who becomes the container for our unbearable painful feelings. When no relief or release from the feelings is obtained, these are re-introjected in their un-digested form and the need to expel feeling even worse is greater, thus expulsion and re-enactments are more and more violent and destructive in order to preserve the self. In the group we strive to put words to experiences and seek to understand and accept the resultant behaviour. This helps to reduce the fear and realise that emotions and feelings can be controlled and contained and together we can learn how to survive this pain.

The group became more used to and accepting of this sharing and holding in the sessions. There are still spills out into the wider community, where they are more easily mopped up and held.

The group membership became more stable, with the majority being life sentence prisoners who could stay in therapy for an extended period of time. They became more able to tolerate and allow for regression and exploration of the more primitive aspects of the self. The regressive pull of group is a well-known phenomenon; the group as a whole reverberates with the resonance of shared feelings. When this 'hits' on the uncontained two-year-old and the terror and rage in all of them finds voice, the result is explosive. This is frightening, especially as the toddlers are now over six foot tall. Over a series of sessions I had been challenging one man for his continued rule breaking and testing the boundaries to the limit. He would not get away with this behaviour on release from prison. The group had held back from this as they had experienced confrontation and hostility from this man before. He raged at me, pinning my ears back and pounding me with his words for several groups. I had a nightmare of being chased down a corridor by the friend of this man. He held me up against the wall and slashed my face down my cheek. I knew that the friend had been set up to do this, unable to face me and express his rage directly. In reality he and his co-defendant had kidnapped and tortured his victim before killing him; the 'victim' was a paedophile who had abused him as a child. I knew of the details of the offence yet this intrusion into my dreams was not usual. I had wakened my partner with sounds of panic and fighting/ kicking in my sleep. This disturbance was too much. As a child I used to sleepwalk, usually when tensions were high in the home. I knew that something was going to come to a head in the group. I had been unaware of why I had chosen to restate the boundaries of the group at this time. I am more active in the group when new members join but not usually in between these events. There was a great sense of threat in the air and my countertransference reaction in behaving uncharacteristically and reinforcing my authority at this point triggered feelings in the group of being trapped in a terrifying situation with the threat of violation. The man who was involved with me in this battle was then challenged by another in the group who was also raped as a boy. There had always been animosity between this pair and it was only now that the malignant mirror was visible to each. They did not choose to fight against me, instead they identified with each other, they could see both their own victim and perpetrator in each other. This resulted in a tremendous discharge of emotions and feelings in a vicious exchange of profanities. There was no relief from this and no escape. The risk of violence was imminent.

The adage of 'trust the group to come up with a solution' sounds great in theory. In practice, in this group, not so. I knew that I was the symbolic but not the direct target for these men and found myself standing between them when they both decided to leave their chairs and get ready to fight each other. The reactions of the other men in the group were interesting; some pulled chairs away and removed themselves from the circle of the group – fear had set off the flight response in them. Others looked ready to fight if need be to avoid being hurt and a couple stood with me in the middle, talking and calming the two combatants. The situation was brought under control. Surviving this to allow them to know that they can be contained without breaking the container or destroying the group or me is healing. They both needed to be able to stand up to each other and before me and not be destroyed or destroy in the process. Neither of them could attack me, the one who symbolised the betrayer of power and control directly. I was also aware that my position of 'sacrifice' to protect them touched the abandoned child within all of us, paralysed with fear and dread. They were stopped from abusing each other and not punished by me. It would have been easier to have just let them bash each other and be discharged from the prison. But that would not have served them well or the group, who would have failed them at the point of maximum distress and pain. As in all trauma therapy, the powerful emotions are often re-visited to be survived again and again until understood to become part of the history rather than the driving force in the current life story. The group had been disabled by the vibrant and explosive content and needed space to allow for the adaptation and moulding of the contents so that both the container and its contents could grow.[5]

The group called a 'special' to give us extra time to sit together as a group and feed back how we each saw and experienced this event. Processing required honesty from me as well. I said that I felt frightened and intimidated and that I thought that was how they felt too. In a less mature group they would have left me to contain all these negative feelings but my disclosure enabled them to own their feelings too. These men are often terrified of their own rage – they killed when in this situation before. The battle to survive and fear of death was a reality for them. Surviving this sort of experience in the group without damage is different; they don't have to kill or be killed any more. For me to stay calm and not retaliate or run away is not difficult. I never did learn when to run! However, maintaining a healthy respect for the dangerousness of the situation is required. I never deny myself the right to feel my own fear as well as theirs. To ignore this would place me in danger. Following this group, I sought out the solace of people I trust and rely on to let me cry and express my fear.

Sitting in the blue corner when the rest are seeing red

I have mentioned briefly the pecking orders in groups and the changes in activity level of the conductor. The following is an example of how changes to the membership affect these groups and how the resultant issues are resolved. The loss of members and each new addition upsets and alters the dynamic of the group. There is a pressure to keep up the number of inmates in the prison, therefore there is little or no time to mourn a loss before the next man comes along. We do attend to planned endings and what it means to move on when we can; however, there are times when the ending is abrupt (e.g. 'ghosting' for drug abuse/dealing) and the change is less manageable. New members in the group are particularly vulnerable to attack, as they upset the status quo and remind others of new arrivals in the family and themselves when they were new to the group. If they had an easy induction they are kinder and more empathic to new members; if not they can take pleasure in giving them the pain that they suffered as the new boy. This is also the time to shift from a position assigned by the group if it no longer feels right to the individual or they wish to have their differing status recognised. There is pride in being the longest member of the group. The displeasure at having the group disrupted and having no control over this often results in scapegoating of the new member. They rarely direct this at me, as they are aware that this is how the community operates, and there is a predominant positive transference towards me as 'their special facilitator' and everything that I represent, whether real or wished for. It can be difficult to draw the transference onto me if I feel it to be necessary, particularly if they have a target in sight and are all fired up. It has taken much time to encourage the group to own their own projections of and to look at what they dislike in another and consider it as a disowned part of themselves. They hate being reminded of these parts of self: 'When I hear you talk I think of what a prat I must have been.'

Joining a group is extremely threatening and the vulnerabilities soon become visible to all. When under threat the men often understandably adopt a narcissistic stance. The difference here is that some have been fighting the whole world and have kicked up against society for as long as they can remember. Some therefore choose to attack the whole group. There have been times when dealing with loss and then having a 'problem child' join the group the container is a bit wobbly and the group as a whole retaliates. Projective identification is rife in this situation, as all have a hook to hang something on. We get into the 'shoot first and ask questions later' scenarios. As the conductor, I had to intervene to prevent the total destruction and annihilation of the individual and the group. The vulnerable, quickly regressed new man projects out all his primitive rage and fear and as a result disrupts and fragments the group. One man was so persistent in his endeavour to beat the therapy (before it got him) that it was impossible to draw the transference completely from him; to take the heat out of the situation I had no option but to side with him. To stick up for him and present things from his perspective and get into his shoes, climb into his corner of the ring with him whilst at the same time keeping a grip on the ropes to take the flak and the heat out of the situation. This experience of having seven angry men having a go put me in a position of complete terror and fear of pain and brutalisation that made death seem like a healthier option. I could see them in a different light, I now knew what it was like to be their victim.

This, of course, is what the isolated new man needed me to know, his experience of terror and his deep fear and mistrust in the group and therapeutic process. His familial experience of being beaten and terrorised by his father was replayed for all to see. Those who have been badly abused can experience the therapy as abusive, especially when defences are penetrated before they are ready and able to withstand the blows. The group does not maintain the attack on me for long and they know that no grudges are held against them. Understanding what just went down takes weeks to unravel and can only be done when they are receptive and ready to hear and reflect on the experience. They struggle to recognise their own abusiveness and enjoy revenge. This scenario also had the effect of sealing a bond between the new man and me. He was protected! Something that his mother did not or could not do. This new experience is appreciated and is one that lasts beyond the therapy. It is also a tremendous test of the conductor that, if failed, results in a repeated empathic failure, lack of trust and a drop-out from the group.

Getting the group out of my head and my body – rape and other violations

So far I have been discussing the part of aggression and violence in the therapy experience. What is often more difficult are their sexual experiences. For many, these were abusive. There are less inhibitions when talking about glassing someone in the face, stabbing or shooting someone or burning down a factory. When it comes to sex, a more intimate and personal encounter, this is treated differently by the group. Exposure to sex and normal sexual development for them was often interfered with either through witnessing sexual acts in the home, rape, buggery, pornographic videos, or being sexualised at an early age through violation and abuse of boundaries from adults and/or peers/ siblings. Mothers figure heavily in the early distortion of their sexual development. Many observed their mothers being dominated and denigrated by their father or other male figures in the family, thus it would appear that their power and expression of sexuality is a threat that needs to be controlled. Sexual acts become split off from attraction and intimacy and kept separate. Sex and violence go hand in hand for many of these men, and few have managed to sustain an intimate sexual relationship, one based on mutual respect and a sharing of pleasure and joy in each other. Early bonds with their mother were often non-existent or destroyed. Thus the longing for a mirroring response to the sexual aspects of self were thwarted during the formative years. An erotic transference develops towards the therapist in this scenario.[6] Some have lots of sex but no intimacy, most will admit to domestic violence, some even though not convicted of sexual offences will admit to the abuse of sexual power. Sexual partners may be seen as objects of sexual gratification, or represent a place to forcefully discharge and displace their own unwanted feelings of violation, powerlessness, inadequacy, disgust, humiliation, denigration and pain. As in violent outbursts, they can dissociate from the victim and fail to empathise with their position. They may enjoy witnessing the other experiencing their split-off and disavowed feelings and emotions. They take control and do what was done to them. They run the risk of enjoying the relief and pleasure that this brings and become addicted to their deviant sexual behaviour. The eroticisation of their primitive libidinal and aggressive feelings is acted out in their sexual behaviour.

The closer and more exposed they become in relationships, the more powerful their defences against feelings of loss of face, failure and inadequacy. This level of intimate contact needs to be within their control and power, most especially if they have been abused. Yet there is something powerfully attractive in these men; they project the image of the potent, strong, powerful male. However, this is often a false self and they are easily crushed and shamed if their sexual potency and prowess is challenged.

The rules of therapy and prison prohibit abuse of the men in engaging in sexual relationships. This does not prohibit the exploration of sexual feelings, flirtatious behaviour and sexual fantasies within the therapeutic relationship. All observed behaviours come back onto the group for discussion. In this way boundaries are held and the re-enactment of incest in the family and the power of secrets, abuse and lies are challenged.

They are often embarrassed to acknowledge their sexual feelings, whether they be to do with lust, love or rape. 'Their self esteem has become organised around the ability to evoke a sexual reaction in others, rather than around non sexual personal attributes. Their demand for love and sexual fulfilment emerges as a "sexualised substitute" for non sexual mirroring of the self that was not sufficiently internalised over the course of development.'[6] This type of disclosure would also give the object of their desires power over them. At times they are like adolescents in their fear of ridicule from others and view their loving feelings as soft and pathetic. When they fall in love they tend to keep this secret. Rape fantasies with women in powerful positions abound in the community, particularly with the female officers who lock them up at night and have control over them. I have to keep my sexual feelings in check constantly. To allow myself to be seduced or to seduce them would create an unhealthy merger and would be disastrous for their development through the therapeutic process. My sexual feelings are explored and worked through in supervision. This transference provides a rich source of meaning of what the eroticised feelings represent. The group tends to hold me in a 'Madonna' position where the power of the mother, symbolic and real, to have compassion, hope for them and set limits as a moral force is what seems to be important to them. Lust does get in the way at times and it is difficult to work with someone when there is a strong sexual attraction as this can get in the way of seeing them for themselves. The men learn to hold the sexual boundaries for themselves, too, and in situations where they find themselves being 'groomed' to in some way satisfy a need of another, they can stop this before they are taken advantage of. They learn to trust their intuitions and stop the violation of the intimate self. Those who perpetually groom their victims repeat this on the wing and in the group. The behaviour is regularly challenged as it is ultimately self-destructive as well as damaging to the object. It leaves those who have been molested or taken in feeling disgusting and dirty for being taken advantage of yet again. Rage and a wish to name, shame and seek revenge is the most common reaction to this type of behaviour. We are all capable of such forms of abuse; few will acknowledge that part of us for fear of this reaction. The fear that some may 'get off on' hearing others' stories of being abused makes it difficult to talk about without feeling that they have been further abused. This highlights the confusion within the individual if their body reacted to the sexual stimulation and they had pleasurable sensations during early sexual abuse.

One of my most disturbing dreams symbolised forced penetration. In the dream I wakened to find my left arm covered in a sheath of composted manure with lots of little seedlings growing out of it. I could not scrape it off, felt uncomfortable, disgusted, felt sick, my skin crawled and I was confused. I was filled with dread and thought that this was a mad dream. I knew, however, that there must be some meaning and that I would have to bear this madness for some reason. Within the week one man talked of his experience of being drugged and anally raped by several men as a child. The dream had been forced into me prior to the telling of his story and allowed me to get in touch with the feelings of dread, disgust, disbelief, confusion, despair, powerless, impotence, annihilation, and shame. The group fell into silence. Some had been convinced this man had been 'blagging' about being abused as an excuse for his behaviour. Now they had to hear the full story, they were shocked, but all believed. No one knew how to respond or react in a helpful way to him. I was able to use some of the words that I had used to describe my dream to myself in supporting him to tell his story. It was a most harrowing experience for all to listen to and be part of. I could empathise with him through the awareness that he had given me. I could also understand the group mirroring the numbness of the shock as my dream had been disturbing and alien to my experiences. This was what he needed me to know to be able to help him to bear the pain of this horrible event which was, of course, totally alien and abhorrent to him. There is always a sense of knowing whom you can tell your most awful secrets to without destroying the relationship. If I had not been accessible to his unconscious communication to me and willing to work with it, it is doubtful that he would have been able to work on this deep and painful memory. The group struggled to hear this story yet were able to listen and to be there in support of this man over the next few days when he was most raw and vulnerable. They treated him with care and respect. Through being contained in this way his most awful wound had been cleansed and the healing could take place.

The mature group – the hall of shame

When the group is fairly settled and cohesive, there is a sense of safety and trust which allows them to work on deeper issues. They can respond to each other with greater care and compassion than before. They are tough on challenging behaviour that is offensive to others but are soft on the person. They are able to pick up, work with and grow the healthy part of each other. The damaged parts are discarded or repaired through the internalisation of the therapy experience. For many it is their maladaptive defences that they no longer require to protect themselves that goes. In the past they learned how to fight but not how to protect themselves; now they learn how to protect without having to fight. The time here in therapy represents the longest adult relationship most of these men have ever had. They experience what it is like to be loved, respected and cared for and they learn to do this for others. Strong bonds and attachments develop, healthy bonds which will sustain them through their life beyond the therapy.

When the group is in this phase, defences come down and the most powerful of all emotions can be shared and talked about. Shame, beyond the last layer of defence in groups.[7] It is rarely talked about in the way observed in this example.

The theme of identity, who you are now and how you were known in the past, emerged following one man's home visit as part of resettlement. Being able to hold your head up, to be answerable for your actions without glorifying them, to be humble but not devastated, was viewed and appreciated as an achievement by those listening. This was heartening to observe. The possibility of change from the who and what of the past is reflected time and time again in the group; they like to see how far they have progressed and praise themselves for this. They each began to speak of their offences and the impact of these on their many victims. They shared the views others presented of them in their witness statements and how they perceived these comments now as opposed to at the time of their trials. Some were shocked by what others had written, some were angry, some rationalised and picked holes in what they read. 'Witness statements' – were they fact or did others build upon the knowledge they had to air grievances long carried or to go along with the 'public' influence and pressure and put them away for a long time?

They moved on to talk of the photographs taken of their victims and the scene of the offence openly with the group. Some had not kept these, refusing to carry them around and risk another inmate seeing them, some chose to erase this factual account. For those with little memory of the actual event, the photographs were a shock to them and the images were now burned into their memories for eternity. Here were the facts, the reality of which could not be doubted or questioned; it happened and they were responsible. Some, the newer and more defended members of the group, did not share, they listened, knowing their own picture was just as gruesome as the next man. The group had taken on the role of bearing witness to the horror of each other's offences. Each having to bear their own feelings of shame, disgust, horror, repulsion, despair and violation. 'Let's face it, if we were shown these pictures and they were of our loved ones, our kids and family, we would be outraged and want to hang us too,' said one man, who had been unable to talk of the full extent of the injuries inflicted by his hand. Owning this and acknowledging that it was they who did this is a huge step for each man, who sits today exposed and vulnerable, open to judgement in the eyes of the harshest critics they will ever find – their mirrors and their own self in the group. No one attacked, no one said it wasn't so bad, all knew how bad the pictures of carnage and destruction were. They were beginning to integrate and tolerate those parts of themselves that they had hated and disowned for so long. Together as a group they were working on their feelings of shame and how they tried to avoid being shamed further by their victims.

What was most striking was how many of them had destroyed or damaged the faces of their victims. They were unable to recognise or even discern the faces; after the attack it could have been anyone or anything. They talked of feeling sick when they looked at these pictures. Some knew their victim, who for various reasons became the focus and repository for all the displaced feelings and emotions pent up from the past and discharged all at once. For others, the victim happened to fit the bill as symbolic or representative of the intended victims. They could not have the face of a real person staring back at them; to have the horror of what they had done mirrored back to the self was unbearable until now. Something had triggered their murderous rage at the time of the offence. Most lost control in the heat of the moment. Some dissociated completely from their victim, unable to see them as a person whilst they carried out a planned attack. At that point they were unable to see beyond the situation. Either they could not identify with the victim or they did with the intention of killing themselves too. Their victims were treated as objects, just as they were as the victims of persistent abuse, ridicule, humiliation and denigration. All of this was projected onto the victim and acted out in a most sadistic and violent way. They found it hard to believe that they were capable of this and were afraid of themselves. They could now see that part of them that was vulnerable, uncontained, unintegrated, uncontrolled and contorted. Their protective image, engineered to defend against all the intolerable emotions and feelings within, was gone. They could now see who and what they truly were when they committed their offence. They talked of the shock and disbelief in their families who had not thought them capable of this; they themselves were shocked by their own action. They could see themselves as aggressors, yet today, at the same time, empathise with their own internal shocked victim.

Facing these demons and looking upon these haunting images had to be done to enable them to move on from the death trap which engulfed them. To stop the hatred and destruction of all feelings and emotions and choose to live a life and incorporate this part of their story requires a major shift. The group as a whole has a greater capacity to bear this intensity of feeling without being defaced or destroyed. This experience of baring emotions and feelings can then be internalised as they each learn to live with their shame. I chose not to say much in this group; I let them talk and share. I did not spell out the gory bits in the feedback to staff, possibly because I would have broken down and cried, struggling to bear this pain with the men, wanting to protect my colleagues from their horrible deeds and wanting to protect the group from further shame. I reacted as they and their families did; sitting with them, I could not bring myself to picture them inflicting such damage and destruction. I felt disabled and too frightened to believe in or express my feelings of despair at the destruction.

'He is a good lad really,' his mother would say on family day. Denying the darker side of us all. We no longer had to deny it and it was no longer secret and no longer filling up a dark space that overshadowed everything that was good.

Vicarious traumatisation of group members and the conductor

'Vicarious traumatisation is the transformation in the inner experience of the therapist that comes about as a result of empathic engagement with clients' trauma material.' 'We do not blame our clients for our experience of vicarious traumatisation. Rather we view it as an occupational hazard, an inevitable effect of trauma.'[1]

What makes me good at what I do is also my curse. The permeability of my internal boundaries which allows free access for unconscious communications from the men helps greatly in understanding them and what is going on between us. This can, however, leave me in a mad and vulnerable space which takes its toll. 'While it is often essential to their healing for clients to share specific traumatic images, we can carry those with us and they may at times appear to us, unbidden, as clear as our own internal images.'[1]

Pressure on the conductor and group to hold something that for the individual is unbearable and with a group that resonates with the same unbearable feelings can be overwhelming. I am usually aware of something being too much for me if I find myself hiding behind the therapist stance or 'lose it' and give an interpretation at the wrong level or withdraw into silence and do not help the group. When this happens the men argue and fight and leave the room. Absences from the group occur. Sweets are shared between the members. These are all signs of my emerging fragility, the group in distress and the risk of the container breaking looms again. We occasionally have what the group calls a 'time of the month group' where we sit together and clear the air of all the things that are troubling them about each other. Their sensitivity to me on an unconscious level is astounding as these groups occur when I am premenstrual and at one level they pick up on my vulnerability. It would be extreme folly to undertake this type of work without one's own prior personal therapy. I regularly see myself in a million pieces in this group; maintaining my integrity can be difficult. The need for regular supervision is paramount, too, as the new 'traumas' experienced from working with this group need to be processed and worked through in the same way as old traumas. Without this I would not be able to be present in the group. The learning from this work is continuous; the homogeneity of a typical outpatient group or a training group does not prepare for this. Generally, life experiences are less extreme, although our ghosts contain many of the aspects of these men in an attenuated or fantasy form. Most are shielded from the rawness of life and death experiences, extreme terror, torture, despair and madness by the experiences that mitigate against the toxic nature of these events – security, love, care, compassion and being comforted and reassured.

It may be that these men have developed a greater capacity or tolerance of these events than they are given credit for. They have borne their own pain and survived. They now develop the capacity to hold onto their feelings that have been made safer and less dangerous in therapy. They learn to control their impulses. However, the total awareness and understanding and acknowledging responsibility for their offence comes at a price. They know that they are no better than their own perpetrators. This feeds guilt and shame and they run the risk of wanting to kill the bad object, the self, totally. They can become very suicidal, dropped back in the loop that got them into trouble before. Holding this fear and anxiety is a tremendous risk for all concerned. This often results in a heavy depression. Klein would say this was progress, but only if able to be held. When I experience deep, dark depression in the countertransference I know that it is time for great care with the men. It is time to listen to and take care of my own mental hygiene too. 'Unaddressed vicarious traumatisation manifest in cynicism and despair, results in a loss to society of that hope and the positive action it fuels. This loss can be experienced by our clients, as we at times join them in their despair; by our friends and families, as we no longer interject optimism, joy and love into our shared pursuits; and in the larger systems in which we are were once active as change agents, and which we may now leave, or withdraw from emotionally in a state of disillusionment and resignation.'[1]

Why do this work, you may ask. As a traumatised teenager I detested those who did not help or understand me when I struggled with my own fears and confusion. I wanted to put things right and offer the kind of support that I never had. I learned how to accept and tolerate all parts of myself, to love myself through my own experience of therapy. I survived and grew as a result of being held. I want others to have that experience too. If they can bear to tell their story, I can bear to listen and share my being with them. I enjoy watching them grow and change, and finally leave therapy, no longer dependent on others for whatever was lacking but able to stand proud and enter life with something we don't often get, another chance to survive and live it to the full.

The emotional cost in this work is high but the rewards to me are priceless.

References

1   Pearlman LA and Saakvitne KW (1995) *Trauma and the Therapist: countertransference and vicarious traumatisation in psychotherapy with incest survivors.* WW Norton Professional, New York.
2   Tuttman S (1994) Therapeutic responses to the expression of aggression by members in groups. In: *Ring of Fire: primitive affects and object relations in group psychotherapy.* Routledge, London.

3   Gartner RB (1999) *Betrayed as Boys: psychodynamic treatment of sexually abused men*. Guilford Press, New York.

4   Gordon J (1994) Bion's post-Experiences in Groups thinking on groups: a clinical example of –K. In: *Ring of Fire: primitive affects and object relations in group psychotherapy*. Routledge, London.

5   Hinshelwood RD (1994) Attacks on the reflective space: containing primitive emotional states. In: *Ring of Fire: primitive affects and object relations in group psychotherapy*. Routledge, London.

6   Stacy CS (1999) Psychic conflict and developmental deficit in the erotically charged transference. Paper presented at APA Division 39 Spring Meeting, New York. http://psychematters.com/papers/stacy.htm

7   Agazarian Y and Peters R (1981) *The Visible and Invisible Group*. Routledge & Kegan Paul Ltd, London.

Chapter 8

Responding to injustice: working with angry and violent clients in a person-centred way

Gillian Proctor

Introduction

In this chapter, I explore the interface between mental health and criminal justice systems from the context of working as a clinical psychologist in forensic services within the NHS mental health system. I explore the problems within the current system and argue that mental health services need to focus clearly on the needs of the distressed individual and leave policing and dealing with violence or harm to others to the criminal justice system. Within the current coercive and policing system, the power relations involved seriously limit the potential for empowering therapeutic work with clients. I explore the relation of anger to the experience of powerlessness, both materially (structurally) and psychologically (in relation to trauma). I argue for the necessity of working therapeutically in a way that does not compound the powerlessness already experienced by the client. To translate this principle into practice, I explain how person-centred therapy (PCT) minimises the chances of the client experiencing further powerlessness in the therapy relationship. I describe how I try to work with this model with clients in forensic services whilst balancing my responsibilities to my clients and to protecting the public. I describe the potential benefits of working using person-centred therapy (PCT), both to the individual clients and to those around them. Finally, I set out the limitations of these benefits caused by the conflict of interests in the current system.

Throughout this chapter, I illustrate my arguments using two potential clients as examples (from an imaginative conglomeration of clinical experience in this setting with a variety of people). These are somewhat stereotypical but illustrate common experiences of clients I have worked with in forensic services. The first, whom I shall call Debbie, is a woman with a history of violence to others, in addition to a history of self-injury. She came to forensic mental health services after setting fire to a chair in a hostel and being diverted from prison due to her psychiatric history and vulnerability. The second client, whom I shall name Paul, is a young man with a history of serious violence who has been referred to forensic services after serving a short prison sentence for assault. He also identifies experiencing much anxiety and depression.

The work context

I work within an NHS mental health trust in the forensic services section. In- and outpatient services are provided to clients who are seen to have mental health problems, are believed to be at current risk of committing serious offences (i.e. involving violence or harm to others), have usually committed serious offences in the past and whose offending behaviour is judged to be related to their mental health problems. Blumenthal[1] emphasises the importance of this context for therapy, saying: 'One of the most striking things about working in forensic services is that the practitioner cannot ignore the context in which he/she works. Unlike other contexts in which therapeutic work takes place, the institution is an omnipresent factor in the therapeutic equation.'

Although this is a mental health service designed to provide a range of treatments for mental health problems, the political priorities are issues of risk and public protection. Kurtz[2] describes this almost exclusive preoccupation with assessing and managing risk as a way of dealing with anxieties aroused by this work, and emphasises the counter-therapeutic culture that results. This prioritising of risk is in line with recent government proposals designed to hold health services more and more responsible for people who used to fall under criminal justice systems. This political agenda ignores the huge problems of inaccuracy in risk prediction.[3,4] Cordess[4] argues that these '"health" proposals and services are being hijacked as agents of social control in order to "police" society'.

Health professionals are now required to attend MAPP (Multi Agency Public Protection) probation-organised meetings to assess and manage the risk that the client may pose to the public. We are required by the MAPP regulations to withhold information about these meetings from the client.[5] Whilst providing a range of treatments to help clients with their distress, we are also required to constantly monitor risk to others and take action if we judge risk to have increased. Thus our responsibility is to our client and to the public, our remit being to improve the client's mental health and reduce their antisocial behaviour. The result of the political focus on risk is that the culture of forensic services is one of defensive practice and of secrecy, with 'information' or judgements being shared among workers without the client's consent. Blumenthal[1] describes the 'constant clash of cultures between a system that privileges punishment, containment and control, and health professionals working to a very different agenda of trying to understand the painful troubled lives of people who inhabit these establishments'.

This clash of cultures led to some mental health professionals involved in Debbie's care only being interested in how often she hit people and not wanting to listen to her distress. She was frequently put into a 'de-escalation room' after threatening or behaving violently, with the overt intention of 'calming her down', though this also had the effect of punishing her for her behaviour. Workers were clearly angry at her behaviour and were happy to have the instruments of control at their disposal to punish her with. Workers involved in Paul's care were split between those emphasising his risk to others and wanting anger management interventions, and those wanting to help him with his experiences of anxiety and depression.

The current model of medical and social control

When is anger an issue for mental health services? When someone's anger is causing a problem for other people or distress to the person themselves? This is not clear in practice. Often referrals to mental health services are made because a person is violent and this is a problem for other people who are victims/potential victims of this violence. Both Debbie and Paul were referred in part due to their risk to others and in part due to their own experiences of distress. Referral on the basis of risk to others is justified as a mental health issue by attaching a diagnosis to a person and individualising their reasons to be angry/violent whilst ignoring the context of their violence.

Anger and particularly violence is often more pathologised in groups where anger or violence is not as culturally acceptable, such as women. Female offenders are more likely than male offenders to be judged as 'mad'.[6] However, the relationship between gender and judgement of risk is complicated. Often, expectations of women being gentle and caring can lead to the risk of serious violence being underestimated in women who have committed serious offences. On the other hand, male offenders with mental health problems are more likely to have their distress ignored, as their behaviour is more in keeping with norms of male behaviour. Most professionals doing the diagnosing are judging appropriateness of such anger or violent behaviour by their own experience of cultural norms, usually white, middle class norms. Paul's level of violence was not unusual for a young man growing up in a housing estate where violence was a way to survive. Risk assessments are of course biased by the judgements of workers making these assessments, and particularly when a client's offence provokes emotions in these workers, such as anger or disgust.

The model of anger management in psychiatric services assumes that anger is a negative emotion – a problem. Most approaches to anger management focus on controlling rather than understanding and learning from anger. This approach ignores all the positive aspects of anger: as a legitimate response to a situation, as an emotion that often gives energy and promotes action (which may be action to promote positive change as opposed to violence). As well as meaning distress or grief, anger also means passion, spirit and feeling. Feeling angry indicates aliveness, passion and a sense of caring about the world. Not feeling angry or ever expressing anger could be considered as just as unhealthy or psychologically damaging as expressing anger.

The current approach in mental health represents the expert professional approach – based on the belief in the objectivity of science and research 'evidence'. This approach assumes objective disease categories, discovered by advances in science, which are then identified by the process of diagnosis. This ignores both the social and political imperatives which shaped the history of psychiatry[7,8] and ignores the huge controversies about the validity of psychiatric diagnoses.[9] The current political agenda is of 'evidence-based practice', which will tell us what works for people with various diagnoses, based on predetermined outcomes of what constitutes mental health and symptom reduction. Again, this notion assumes that 'evidence' is objective, thus obscuring the political and economic vested interests involved in what questions are asked in research, in which research is funded and in deciding what research counts as 'evidence'. The notion of 'objectivity' has long been questioned within science itself and yet the mental health system is still based on the myth of value-free 'objective' observers.

Instead, a more accurate description of the process of psychiatrisation or pathologisation of certain areas of human experience is that new categories become the business of mental health as a result of political or media pressures. 'Road rage', for example, arose as a new concept within mental illness as a result of the media focus on the problem of violence whilst driving. The incorporation of this concept into an individualised notion of mental illness suggests that a condition or disease in certain individuals which causes road rage was 'discovered'. Similarly, the diagnosis of 'personality disorder' has become increasingly common in the last decade, in line with the political pressures for mental health to incorporate more of a criminal justice role.[10] This 'expert' and 'objective' research-based model of mental health services makes these services prime targets for social control and political pressures to use treatment to normalise individuals and be agents of social control.

There are always reasons why someone is angry and why they may express this using violence. This may include a complex mix of factors including personal historical experiences and cultural norms which may be more difficult for individuals to articulate. People are often angry as a result of experiences of violation, abandonment, disrespect and injustice. Blumenthal[1] emphasises the optimism of those practitioners, responding to the current political climate by 'viewing offending behaviour as a symptom of a disturbed personality that needs to be understood'. Using offending behaviour as the basis of a diagnosis (usually a type of personality disorder) places the blame for relational and social problems in the individual (individualising societal problems) and leaves little room for understanding complex unique individuals. In addition, individualising and pathologising anger and violence as a disorder has the danger of removing responsibility from individuals for their behaviour. Any 'understanding' needs to be of relational and social experiences and how the individual has responded to these experiences within their socio-political context. In addition, understanding is hard to achieve in a system where workers are also serving the purpose of control and punishment.

Alternative social, psychological and responsibility model of mental health

There have historically been two distinct services – criminal justice services and mental health services. Criminal justice is supposed to deal with people who have been a risk to society due to their behaviour. Mental health is supposed to help individuals with their own needs concerning individual distress. However, it may be more accurate to argue that both systems serve to get rid of people who don't function as society wants them to.[7,8,11,12] The distinction between the two has been blurred for a long time as a result of coercive psychiatric treatment.[12,13]

Here, I am suggesting a (currently) fictional alternative to the current model of medical and social control based on clarity about the distinction between matters of crime and matters of mental distress. Thus, causing harm to others by violence is a matter of crime covered by the criminal justice system. Feeling distressed as a result of the experience of anger or as a result of being violent is a matter for mental health services. Individuals may seek mental health services when they identify difficulties themselves that feeling angry or being violent causes them. These may be *internal* psychological difficulties due to living with such feelings or *relational* social difficulties due to the effect of their anger/violence on others around them. Debbie wanted help due to her internal experience of anger and hurt rooted in the ways she had been treated as a child. Paul identified difficulties relating to others and trusting people as a result of being perceived by others as 'scary'.

Within this alternative model of mental health, the causes of distress are social, and individuals live within social contexts which determine or affect their behaviour. For example, violence is common for people like Paul, a way to survive in certain cultural and social contexts, such as some lower working class housing estates in the UK characterised by unemployment and drug use. He was also angry about both historical and current ways he was treated by others. For Debbie, anger is one common result of experiencing sexual, physical and emotional abuse as a child, having her child taken away from her and her distress being ignored now. In addition, she had learned to express distress through violence from her father's violence towards her. For each person, historical and current, personal relational and wider social factors all combine to both cause anger and influence an individual's choice to be violent. Within this alternative model, services are provided as requested by service users, and service users are trusted to know what is most helpful for them and to determine their own criteria of wellness or happiness.

This model is only possible if individual distress is separated from harm to others. Thus mental health services and therapy are separated from criminal justice and societal control systems. If the two are combined, this means a view of mental health is imposed which includes not being violent and this aim can easily supersede and obscure any aims for the client to feel better themselves. In addition, this aim from outside takes control, power and responsibility away from the individual. For lasting changes within the client, which may include a reduction in violence, the client needs to be in control of this process. Without personal control over this change, the only alternative is to police behaviour by contingencies outside the person. This has historically been the role of the criminal justice system. Paul or Debbie may decide to stop being violent to avoid going to prison but when there is little risk of that, they are likely to still be violent.

When mental health workers have the responsibility for dealing with offending and risk in addition to the mental health needs of the client, the result of this can be that offences are focused on and workers subsequently often identify with the victims of these offences. It is then very difficult for workers to *understand* the client as opposed to feeling angry with them and wanting them to be controlled or punished. Often a cycle is then perpetuated, where workers take more control over clients, who get angrier as a result of their increasing powerlessness. When attempts were made to control Debbie's violence by means of 'de-escalation', she became more and more angry and violent as a result of her increasing frustration.

The socio-political context

People who end up in a forensic mental health service have often come from deprived, oppressive and powerless situations. There is a hugely dispropor- tionate number of men from African and Caribbean ethnic backgrounds within the service.[14] People who enter the forensic service (predominantly men) have often come from circumstances where few choices were available, in particular, choices to increase their social power.

How people express anger varies enormously both individually and depend- ing on structural placing in society, such as gender, ethnicity and particularly class. Indermaur[15] argues that cultural beliefs about anger as well as the purpose and acceptability of violence influence the decision to use violence, which explains cross-cultural and gender differences in the use of violence. Whereas Kring[16] reports that anger is typically a response to threat or to perception of deliberate or unjustifiable harm or negligence, I argue that in addition, anger is often a response to inequities in society and the experience of powerlessness or threat of losing power related to these hierarchies. De Zulueta[17] argues that violence is a result of the power structure of patriarchy, saying 'It is the dehumanisation of the other that is the root of all human violence, a dehumanisation that unfortunately appears almost intrinsic to the development of the male-female sexual role differentiation seen in patriarchal cultures' (p. xiii).

For Paul, violence was a way to survive and not be victimised or humiliated in a context where violence was the currency of everyday relating to others. Violence kept him at the top of a hierarchy by others' fear of him. For Debbie, her anger stemmed from her experiences of extreme powerlessness as a child and as a mother having her child removed, and was triggered by current experiences of being invalidated or ignored, i.e. where her position as a valued human was questioned. For each of them, anger and violence were responses to and a fight against powerlessness.

Schieman[18] examines the effects of education on anger and concludes that differences related to education are explained by the individual's sense of control indicating that the experience of power or powerlessness may be the significant factor explaining structural variations. Brantlinger[19] investigated adolescent behaviour which got them into trouble in school. She found that whereas high-income adolescents reported mainly playful behaviour, low- income adolescents reported more aggressive behaviours likely to have stemmed from anger. These students validated this assumption, describing reasons for their anger including being humiliated and ostracised by high-income students and treated unfairly by teachers. Brantlinger[20] also noted that the low-income adolescents' displays of anger or withdrawal were likely to be perceived by others as signs of emotional disturbance and not as legitimate responses to social class inequities in school and society.

Debbie described a history of failing in school and feeling constantly humiliated for this failure. When she expressed her anger to her parents, she was physically abused under the guise of 'punishment'. Paul also described a history of 'failing' at school. He explained that he had never really learned to read or write properly and had been 'dumped' in the bottom stream in a class where the teachers' priorities were containment as opposed to education. Despite Paul's frustration and boredom at school, his parents encouraged him to just fight and get through time at school until he was old enough to leave. His fighting proved to himself and his peers that he was in the bottom stream due to his bad behaviour and not his inability to learn.

Kring[16] discusses the discrepancy between clinical literature suggesting that women internalise and men externalise anger and experimental research findings that generally do not support this gender difference in the general population. She suggests that there are more similarities than differences in experience of anger in men and women but differences are found in particular contexts. Most differences are found in the experience and expression of anger between men and women in the context of interpersonal relationships. Men report more physical assaults of objects and people and verbal assaults, whereas women cry more often when angry. She reports evidence to suggest that feminine sex-role characteristics are associated with suppressing anger and masculine characteristics are associated with expressing anger in both men and women. Some authors suggest that gender differences in anger expression and experience may reflect variations in power or status more than differences in gender.

Kring[16] suggests that the clinical literature tends to perpetuate the stereotypes of men and women concerning anger expression. Although behaviour tends not to represent these stereotypes, the stereotypes persist, so that although women may readily experience and express anger, they are still judged more than men for doing so. However, there is evidence that within forensic settings women and men experience and express anger differently.[21] The inconsistent findings between women in the general population and women in clinical samples may represent a difference in how women negotiate their sex-role stereotypes. It seems that women who conform strongly or rebel strongly may be over-represented in clinical samples as opposed to 'general population' samples, which have more women who struggle less with their gender-role stereotypes. This may reflect the association of how women negotiate gender-role stereotypes with pathologisation and diagnosis.

Chesler,[22] for example, coined the term 'double-bind' to describe the processes by which women can be pathologised both for conforming to, and for failing to conform to, expectations of feminine passivity. The diagnosis of Borderline Personality Disorder, for example, can be applied to women who fail to live up to their gender role because they express anger and aggression. In addition, the diagnosis is given to women who conform 'too strongly', by internalising anger, and expressing this through self-focused behaviour such as self-injury.[10] The clinical differences may also reflect the association of distress and powerlessness in such settings with how women may use sex-role stereotypes to experience more power. Thus, a situation is set up in clinical settings that reinforces stereotypes of gender roles, leaving these stereotypes more available to women in these settings to use to increase their power.

Much research has been conducted investigating differences in experience and expression of anger depending on structural variables such as gender, ethnicity and social class. This research is consistent with the suggestion that differences in anger expression and experience reflect variations in power or status. This supports my argument that anger and violence is often a response to powerlessness or the threat of losing power. This seems to be a natural consequence of our hierarchical society, where life is a constant competition to stay on top and in order to stay on top, others need to be put down. Another characteristic of this hierarchical system is that those below us are dehumanised, making it easier for them to be the victims of our violence.

Anger and trauma

The experience of anger can be clearly related to the experience of powerlessness additionally through a consideration of the effects of trauma. Anger is one of the common emotional reactions to the experience of trauma. Walsh[23] demonstrated a relationship between exposure to community violence and symptoms of distress and expression of anger in adolescents. De Zulueta[17] argues that violence is a result of the invalidation of our sense of self through deprivation, loss or trauma. Finkelhor[24] identifies four dynamics following the experience of childhood sexual abuse, which include stigmatisation and the experience of powerlessness. Both of these dynamics are related to the experience of dehumanisation. It seems that violence may be the result of fear of vulnerability or the experience of having one's vulnerability taken advantage of.

Powerlessness and psychological distress

I argue that the experience of powerlessness is one of the most significant causal factors contributing to the experience of psychological distress.[25,26] Power, control and the experience of powerlessness are major factors in understanding all kinds of psychological distress. I also argue that the higher prevalence of members of oppressed groups in mental health systems reflects the positions of power of the groups involved.[25,26] There is much evidence to associate the likelihood of suffering from psychological distress with the individual's position in society with respect to societal structural power. When mental health professionals ignore the links between social inequalities and psychological distress, they serve the interests of privileged social groups rather than those of their clients. As Smail[27] states, clients of the mental health system are 'people upon who the world has impinged in any of a variety of painful ways. They are less people with whom anything is wrong than people who have suffered wrong.' The power of medicalisation and pathologising individuals serves to divert attention from the environmental causes of distress, the experiences of abuse, deprivation and powerlessness. Instead 'disordered' individuals are blamed for society's ills.

Starhawk[28] distinguishes between power-over, power-from-within and power-with. Power-over is domination, coercive authority, the ultimate manifestation being violence. Society is based on structures of power-over within hierarchies where those above have power-over those below. In contrast, power-from-within is an inner strength from a sense of mastery at one's own ability and innate value, which also arises from the sense of connection with other humans and the environment. This is also similar to Rogers' concept of 'personal power'.[29,30]

Power-with is the power of individuals within a group of equals to suggest and be listened to. This is reminiscent of Arendt's concept of power by collectivity and consent. Arendt[31] emphasises the 'enormous potential' in the power of mutuality and people acting together for the benefit of all.* These three aspects of power are interrelated. People have less need to take power-over others when they have a strong sense of power-from-within or power-with. Violence is only necessary when influence fails.

Clearly, the way to deal with difficulties that stem from abuse, deprivation and powerlessness is not to impose further power and control through the psychiatric system. Psychiatric systems are much more successful in controlling people experiencing distress than in helping to alleviate distress. One example of this is the common response to self-injury within psychiatric hospitals, where patients are put on 'observation' to try and prevent self-injury. However, there are rarely interventions to help patients with the underlying distress. Or, when these interventions are in place, patients are often forced to talk to staff, whether they want to or not. We cannot resolve distress (as opposed to policing distress) by taking more power-over people.[25,28] A relationship where an individual's power is not taken away and she/he is treated with respect provides the best chance for people to heal from experiences and develop other ways to feel their own power-from-within rather than having power over others.

Working within the current context

The current medical and social control context of working raises particular difficulties and constraints for practitioners wanting to work in a person-centred way or with ethical frameworks which prioritise client autonomy, control and choice. However, if a person her/himself identifies a problem, I believe it is possible to work phenomenologically from an ethical base within the constraints of the system to enable people to make changes for themselves

---

* See Proctor (2002)[25] for more details about models of power including those of Starhawk and Arendt.

that are likely to result in decreasing their risk to other people. If mental health can be focused on the needs of the individual in their social context, the fortuitous results of that are usually that harm to others is also reduced. When people's needs are met, it seems that they are less likely to hurt others. When people are understood, they are more able to understand others and when people are valued, they are more likely to value others.

Person-centred therapy (PCT)

The results of 40 years of psychotherapy research have consistently discovered the importance of the *quality* of the therapy relationship for effective and good therapy. Summaries of the research outcome studies over the last 35 years[32,33] demonstrate that the effectiveness of psychotherapy depends primarily on the therapy relationship and the inner and external resources of the client. In the majority of cases, the type of therapy, techniques used, training or credentials of the therapist are found to be irrelevant, and the most consistent relationship variables related to effectiveness are empathy, genuineness and unconditional positive regard. The commonalities in successful therapy relationships are consistent with the philosophy and theory of person-centred therapy (PCT).

Rogers methodically examined hours of recorded and transcribed therapy sessions to examine what the ingredients of effective therapy were. The result of this research was the description of six necessary and sufficient conditions of the therapeutic process.[34] He then elaborated this theory of therapy to a theory of personality. He theorised that these conditions of therapy helped the actualising tendency fulfil its full potential and work as well as possible and to counteract conditions of worth.[34] Rogers[35] describes these conditions similarly in his 'integration statement',[32] where he asserts that they are the necessary and sufficient conditions in all therapy.

Person-centred therapy and power

Rogers explicitly set out to change the role of the therapist from that of an expert and to aim for a more egalitarian therapy relationship. This follows from the philosophy underlying person-centred therapy. Rogers[30] contends that the premise of the actualising tendency challenges the need to control people; i.e. challenges:

> 'The view that the nature of the individual is such that he cannot be trusted – that he must be guided, instructed, rewarded, punished, and controlled by those that are higher in status.' (p. 8)

He explains the implications of this philosophy and values:

> 'The politics of the person-centred approach is a conscious renunciation and avoidance by the therapist of all control over, or decision-making for, the client. It is the facilitation of self-ownership by the client and the strategies by which this can be achieved; the placing of the locus of decision-making and the responsibility

for the effects of these decisions. It is politically centred in the client.'[30] (p. 14)

This trust in the client's process leads to the non-directive attitude. The *non-directive attitude* is a way for therapists to express their commitment to avoiding client disempowerment.[36] In this sense PCT is a radical disruption of the dynamics of power in therapy. Natiello[29] (p. 11) explains that, 'Such a stand is in radical conflict with the prevailing paradigm of authoritarian power'. I argue that the aim for the PCT therapist is to reduce 'power-over' the client as far as possible and to maximise the 'power-from-within' of both client and therapist and the 'power-with' in the therapy relationship.[25]

Rogers asserts that opposition to person-centred therapy sprang 'primarily because it struck such an outrageous blow to the therapist's power'[30] (p. 16). He challenges the notion of expert knowledge which gives power, and believes in the knowledge and power that comes from congruence, that:

'In such an individual, functioning in a unified way, we have the best possible base for wise action. It is a process base, not a static authority base. It is a trustworthiness that does not rest on "scientific" knowledge.'[30] (p. 250)

Ethical principles

The fundamental ethical principle behind PCT is of the autonomy of the client as opposed to the moral principle of beneficence (doing what's judged to be best for the client) employed by many other models of therapy. Most people have had too many experiences of being told what to do by others (people taking 'power-over') and too few experiences in being really trusted and helped to decide what is right for themselves (to experience their 'power-from-within'). This is likely to be particularly true of clients in a forensic setting.

Following from the ethical principle of autonomy is the emphasis on informed consent and the openness and honesty of clinicians. Given the many reasons most clients will have to not trust people in authority, these principles give a clinician a good start in providing an unusually honest basis for a relationship in a service which is too often based on secrecy and authority. Paul only agreed to work with me on the basis that he saw everything I wrote in his file including letters to other workers. This was as a result of having had several reports written about him by professionals previously that had been used for legal purposes, that had labelled him with many diagnoses and personal judgements, including being a 'psychopath', and suggested that any kind of treatment or therapy was doomed to failure as there was no hope of him changing.

Process of PCT

Rogers[34,37] describes the process that a client who experiences the facilitative conditions of therapy characteristically goes through. The characteristic outcomes of therapy (as generalisations from research) do not lead to the therapist holding aims for the client but merely describe changes that *are likely* to occur as a result of the facilitative conditions. During the process of therapy, the client is likely to be aware of more of his/her inner experiencing and able to accurately experience more of his/her perceptions. In reciprocity with the attitudes experienced by the therapist towards the client, it is likely that the client increasingly feels positive self-regard, is increasingly free to be his/herself and understands his/herself better. In reciprocity with these changes towards self, the client is also likely to experience more positive regard and understanding of others.

This process could be relevant to clients who are angry in many ways. In the process of more accurately perceiving and understanding inner experiencing, the client is likely to be better at identifying all their feelings in reaction to their experiences. It may be that clients who previously reacted with anger to many experiences are able to differentiate their feelings to a greater extent and identify feelings other than anger, such as hurt, which they previously understood to be anger. As the client feels more congruent and experiences more positive self-regard and empathy, she/he is less likely to distort and deny experiences both in the present and memories of previous experiences. Thus a client who has had experiences leading to anger is likely to be aware of these experiences to a greater extent and thus perhaps experience anger more; however, this anger is more likely to be experienced and understood to be associated with these specific experiences. A client's anger towards her/himself is likely to decrease as positive self-regard increases. Violence towards other people is likely to decrease as the client's understanding and positive regard of others increases.

In the process of PCT, Debbie elaborated her emotions concerning how her family had treated her in the past and how others were currently treating her and communicated much more about how hurt and ashamed she felt in addition to feeling angry. As she explored this in therapy, she became increasingly able to talk to other workers about her distress. She also increased her expression of her sense of injustice about her situation. During Debbie's therapy, she expressed more and more details about the abuse she received as a child, particularly the aspects of these experiences of which she felt most ashamed. She expressed her experience of powerlessness, failure, shame and great pain when her child was taken away. She also became more aware of how current situations had the potential to cause similar emotions to those she had in relation to her childhood experiences. As Debbie explored more about how she was treated as a child and blamed herself for this treatment, she began to challenge this perception more and more and to feel that nothing she had done would lead her to deserve the abuse she received. Over time, Debbie became clearer that the responsibility for her experiences of abuse lay with her abusers. While she tried to understand why her abusers behaved in this way, her anger towards her abusers did not diminish. However, she was more able during the process of therapy to understand the behaviour of others in her current life who annoyed her and disrespected her as not necessarily intentional whilst holding onto her sense of worth as a person.

In the process of PCT for Paul, he thought more about his experiences as a child and how he had been taught to be violent from a young age. He explored how he had begun to use violence to gain power when feeling powerless and to keep others away from him by fear so he felt less vulnerable. As he began to understand himself more, he also started to feel more positive about himself and value his strengths and his ability to adapt to survive. He also became more accepting of his vulnerability and need for others and more open to others about when he felt scared or insecure. As his anxiety and depression had already stopped him being part of the culture he had been part of, he decided to use this opportunity to stop being violent and as his anxiety decreased he felt less need to defend himself in this way. This was difficult for some time due to the difficulty of changing others' perceptions of him and still being part of the same social circle. However, over time, as he became more open about his vulnerabilities, he was able to depend on others more for emotional support and developed closer relationships, which again increased his self-esteem. As he opened up more to others, he found that people close to him did the same with him and he began to find it easier to understand and respect the motivations and behaviours of others.

Difficulties working with PCT with angry/violent clients

Clients seen in a forensic setting are often given as examples of how it must be difficult to keep the attitudinal conditions for the therapist in PCT. Students of PCT often ask: how can you experience unconditional positive regard (UPR) or empathic understanding for a client who has raped or murdered? How can you be congruent if you feel horrified, disgusted or angry about what your client has done or feel free to be yourself if you feel afraid of the client?

I too thought my judgement could be a problem before working in this area. My initial aim was to not judge the person even if I judged the behaviour. However, I found that even if I tried to separate the behaviour and judged *that*, this prevented me from really understanding how the client came to behave that way. Instead, I have found that the more I aim to fulfil the conditions and aim to understand my client without judgement, the more I am actually able to understand the reasons why they have committed the offences they have, and in understanding that I find it very easy not to judge. On occasion I find myself judging aspects of a client's attitudes and then work out in supervision what is preventing me from getting closer to understanding their perspective. So far I have been able to figure out what in my beliefs and experiences prevents me from going further into the perspective of particular individuals. However, even with the client with whom I had the most difficulty under-standing and not judging (actually not in a forensic setting), I was still able to continue to try understanding more with regular supervision and to be with him enough for him to find this valuable despite my clear (to me) deficiencies.

Regarding congruence, on occasion I have felt horrified, angry or disgusted by what clients have told me they have done or have wanted to do, usually when I am identifying with the potential victim rather than my client. Again, supervision has been invaluable for me to share these feelings. When a client is talking about considering doing something to hurt someone else I will certainly express my concern for the potential victim, if worry about the victim is preventing me from trying to be with the client. I then concentrate on trying to understand the complexity of their current experience and if I am still concerned at the end of the meeting that they are likely to do what they are planning, I will discuss my concerns again and decide if I need to inform someone else in line with my limits in confidentiality, of which my clients will already be aware.

Working with Debbie, for some time I found it difficult to understand and accept how she was unable to take responsibility for hurting the people she assaulted. However, over time, her confusion about her lack of responsibility for this whilst being charged by the police became clearer as she explored the links between her current behaviour and her experiences of being hurt as a child and always believing it was her fault and responsibility, due to her behaviour which upset her father.

Particular difficulties working with PCT in a forensic setting

Rather than the nature of the clients themselves in this system or the offences they have committed, my major difficulties in doing PCT are in being part of such a coercive, judgemental, punishing or parentalistic system. The stigma faced by clients who are or have been part of a forensic psychiatry service are immense, for a client is labelled both a criminal (bad) and mad. People in the UK who are moved from prison to a mental health setting are likely to be incarcerated for far longer than if they had stayed in a criminal justice setting, and sometimes with very little more in the way of 'treatment' than would be offered by a standard prison. There are workers attracted to this area because they enjoy the power to control and punish people and take pride in the 'macho' image of this work.

Clients in this system face huge discrimination in terms of employment and housing in addition to their day-to-day decisions of who to trust with what information. Cordess[4] locates people defined as 'criminal' and 'mentally ill' within a long history of being labelled as 'other' and thus stigmatised. These 'others' are then analysed 'not as citizens or even people but as problems to be solved or confined'. This process is reminiscent of the process of dehumanisation of those below us in the hierarchy. Cordess[4] warns that 'greater and greater coercion merely induces greater identification with such coercive methods'. Coercion increases powerlessness, suspicion, mistrust and paranoia in clients and workers alike.

Obviously, within this culture and environment it is very difficult to create an environment of honesty, trust and empowerment within therapy. I am clear with clients and colleagues that I will play no part in clients being coerced to see me, and emphasise their choice in choosing to take part in therapy. However, I cannot always be aware of what other workers have told their clients or how they could have tried to 'persuade' or coerce their clients to see me. Whereas this is always the case in any kind of therapy context regarding other people in the client's life, I need to work harder in this system to give the message of choice to the client and colleagues.

The moral basis of PCT is completely at odds with the general culture of forensic services in the NHS. There, the principles upheld are of distrust of the client and expert professionals whose job it is to protect the public by controlling dangerous clients. The big focus on public protection is often, in my view, prioritised above client care. If the therapist's main concern is to reduce risk and he sees the client as a 'danger', the PCT therapist's attitudes are likely to be much harder to achieve. To be able to work towards these attitudes the therapist must be able to focus on the needs of the client.

The political principles of the service provide severe constraints for the person-centred practitioner, and I strive to be as honest and open as possible with my clients about my role within the system and in particular my additional responsibility for public protection. I am clear about the limits of my confidentiality and when I need to depart from trying to be with and understand the client to asking specifically about risk to others and informing others about these risks. However, thinking of protecting others does take me away at times from being with my client and limits how much I can really be with a client and try and enter into their world, whilst part of me judges from the outside whether I need to assess current risk to others.

My trust in each client's innate potential for positive growth or change (the actualising tendency) does not mean I can trust that the client will not offend or harm others during their process of growth. I certainly cannot predict where that process will take the client, but believe it is the most trustworthy basis for positive change. Ultimately I trust the client's innate tendency towards growth to take them on the most positive path possible for him/herself better than I or anyone else can know what that path could be. I find that the more I respect the autonomy of a client and try and understand their experience, often, the more they are able to work out for themselves why they do the things they have done and take steps to be responsible and stop hurting others. Even if they are unable to take this responsibility, often within the context of our relationship, they are willing to give me the information necessary to act and prevent danger to themselves or others.

Worral[38] describes this as follows:

> '. . . [Empathy] demands critical intelligence as well as emotional sensitivity, head as well as heart. It demands that we trust the process of actualisation and at the same time that we process the trust, critique it, so that we trust with our eyes open. In this way, it carries the philosophy of the person-centred approach and makes a legitimate space for the optimism of the approach in a world which is often more cynical than optimistic.'

I have also learned from experience the importance of clarity regarding the difference between *understanding* someone's feelings of anger or desire to hurt another and *acting* on the basis of someone's plans to do so immediately. I act within PCT when I try and understand someone's feelings and then may need to clarify if I also have a public protection duty to act upon. At times, it is not clear if clients are expressing their feelings of anger towards people (which would require PCT), or if they are declaring their intentions to hurt others (which would require my action to inform someone). At these times, I clarify with clients the meaning of their communications and whether there is any intent for action.

Conclusion

Anger and violence are human experiences that need to be understood within the cultural context of each individual. Working with angry people within forensic services raises many difficulties as a result of the social and political context of the system. The issue of power pervades the system within which I work and the dual aims of treatment and control are often opposed. Working in forensic services with the person-centred approach is a constant challenge. This culture makes my approach even more essential to try and provide a more empowering experience for clients. I find this work is possible if I identify myself firmly with my client and try to be there for their needs.

However, in my ideal mental health system, I would be able to provide a more effective and empowering service for clients experiencing difficulties with anger.

Working ethically with clients who are experiencing anger necessitates clarity about who has the problem. Mental health services need to be set up with the priority of reducing distress, leaving policing and public protection to the criminal justice system. Only if we leave the problems of violence hurting others to the criminal justice system can mental health services give angry clients like Debbie and Paul the consideration they deserve, without assuming the necessary negativity of anger and trying to understand experiences rather than condemn or control.

References

1 Blumenthal S (2002) Editorial: violence and its institutions. *Criminal Behaviour and Mental Health.* **12**(2): S1–S4.
2 Kurtz A (2002) A psychoanalytic view of two forensic mental health services. *Criminal Behaviour and Mental Health.* **12**(2): S68–S80.
3 Zigmond A (2002) Mental health legislation – my patients and me. *Make up your Mind* – conference on the Reform of Mental Health Law and Mental Incapacity.
4 Cordess C (2002) Proposals for managing dangerous people with severe personality disorder: new legislation and new follies in a historical context. *Criminal Behaviour and Mental Health.* **12**(2): S12–S19.
5 Home Office (2000) *Criminal Justice and Court Services Act 2000.* TSO, London.
6 Burns J (1992) Mad or just plain bad? Gender and the work of forensic clinical psychologists. In: J Ussher and P Nicolson (eds) *Gender Issues in Clinical Psychology.* Routledge, London.
7 Foucault M (1977) *Discipline and Punish.* Penguin Press, London.

8   Foucault M (1977) *Madness and Civilisation*. Tavistock, London.
9   Boyle M (1999) Diagnosis. In: C Newnes, G Holmes and C Dunn (eds) *This is Madness: a critical look at psychiatry and the future of mental health services*. PCCS Books, Ross-on-Wye.
10 Shaw C and Proctor G (2004) Hidden agenda: a critique of borderline personality disorder. *Asylum* (in press).
11 Pilgrim D (1987) *Psychotherapy and Society*. Sage, London.
12 Szasz T (1997, first published 1970) *The Manufacture of Madness: a comparative study of the inquisition and the mental health movement*. Syracuse University Press, Syracuse, NY.
13 Newnes C and Holmes G (1999) The future of mental health services. In: C Newnes, G Holmes and C Dunn (eds) *This is Madness: a critical look at psychiatry and the future of mental health services*. PCCS Books, Ross-on-Wye.
14 Fernando S (1991) *Mental Health, Race and Culture*. Macmillan/MIND, London.
15 Indermaur D (1999) Perceptions of violence. *Psychiatry, Psychology and Law*. 3(2): 129–41.
16 Kring A (2000) Gender and anger. In: A Fischer (ed.) *Gender and Emotion: social psychological perspectives*. Cambridge University Press, Cambridge.
17 De Zulueta F (1993) *From Pain to Violence: the traumatic roots of destructiveness*. Whurr, London.
18 Schieman S (2000) Education and the activation, course, and management of anger. *Journal of Health and Social Behavior*. 41(1): 20–39.
19 Brantlinger E (1993) Adolescents' interpretation of social class influences on schooling. *Journal of Classroom Interaction*. 28(1): 1–12.
20 Brantlinger E (1991) Social class distinctions in adolescents' reports of problems and punishment in school. *Behavioural Disorders*. 17(1): 36–46.
21 Suter JM, Byrne MK, Byrne S *et al.* (2002) Anger in prisoners: women are different from men. *Personality and Individual Differences*. 32(6): 1087–100.
22 Chesler P (1972) *Women and Madness*. Doubleday, New York.
23 Walsh M (1995) The relationship of exposure to community violence with post-traumatic stress disorder and expression of anger in adolescents. *Dissertation Abstracts International*. 56(5-A): 1988.
24 Finkelhor D (1986) *A Sourcebook on Child Sexual Abuse*. Sage, London.
25 Proctor G (2002) *The Dynamics of Power in Counselling and Psychotherapy: ethics, politics and practice*. PCCS Books, Ross-on-Wye.
26 Proctor G (2002) Therapy in the NHS: who's got the power? *Healthcare Counselling and Psychotherapy Journal*. 2(4): 26–9.
27 Smail D (1987) Psychotherapy as subversion in a make-believe world. *Changes*. 4(5): 398–402.
28 Starhawk (1987) *Truth or Dare: encounters with power, authority and mystery*. Harper and Row, San Francisco.
29 Natiello P (2001) *The Person-centred Approach: a passionate presence*. PCCS Books, Ross-on-Wye.
30 Rogers CR (1978) *Carl Rogers on Personal Power*. Constable, London.

31 Arendt H (1986) Communicative power. In: S Lukes (ed.) *Power*. Basil Blackwell, Oxford.

32 Bozarth J (1998) *Person-centred Therapy: a revolutionary paradigm*. PCCS Books, Ross-on-Wye.

33 Paley G and Lawton D (2001) Evidence-based practice: accounting for the importance of the therapeutic relationship in UK National Health Service therapy provision. *Counselling and Psychotherapy Research*. **1**(1): 12–17.

34 Rogers CR (1959) A theory of therapy, personality and interpersonal relationships as developed in the client-centred framework. In: S Koch (ed.) *Psychology: a study of a science, Vol. III: Formulations of the Person and the Social Context*. McGraw-Hill, New York and London.

35 Rogers CR (1957) The necessary and sufficient conditions for therapeutic personality change. *Journal of Consulting Psychology*. **21**: 95–103.

36 Brodley BT (1997) The non-directive attitude in client-centered therapy. *The Person Centered Journal*. **4**(1): 18–30.

37 Rogers CR (1961) *On Becoming a Person: a therapist's view of psychotherapy*. Constable, London.

38 Worral M (2001) Supervision and empathic understanding. In: S Haugh and T Merry (eds) *Rogers' Therapeutic Conditions: evolution, theory and practice. Vol. 2: Empathy*. PCCS Books, Ross-on-Wye.

Chapter 9

Violence, sexual offending and sexual abuse: are they linked? A qualitative research study

Michael Parker

Introduction

In Canada, sexual offences have been included within the legal framework of violent offences and Canadian Law uses the term 'aggravated sexual assault' in place of the term 'rape'.[1] This was done in recognition of the powerful impact of sexual assault on the victims of this particular crime. This law effectively dissolves the distinction between the two offences and equates sexual offending with violence or assault. In the UK the two offences are still judged under different statutes. What is similar in effect between the two offences is personal violation of the victim assaulted and the frequent subsequent emotional and psychological trauma experienced by victims of both crimes. This chapter looks at sexual offending as a perverse expression of violence occurring within an attachment disorder.

Currently, high profile media attention is paid to sexual crimes, since their occurrence is more commonly reported and known about. Attention tends more towards the issue of punishment and sentencing of sexual offenders, while any understanding of why such a crime should be committed remains in the background. At the present time it appears difficult to include any substantial public understanding of this offence, because it is at such a pitch of unpopularity. Sexual crimes such as paedophilia have in the past remained more hidden and often undiscovered or unreported, due perhaps to factors such as fear or shame in disclosing the facts of sexual abuse. It may still be early in the process of digesting the implications of this crime for more understanding of its origins to be woven into the process of media or professional discussion. However, largely omitted in current dialogue is any exploration of the life history of sexual offenders as a clue to the meaning or purpose of these acts and this chapter addresses itself to any such possible meaning.

Current sexual abuse research literature

Fattah points to a link between victims and perpetrators of crime in his general theory of victimology.[2] His finding of a link between victims and perpetrators of crime may have an intrapersonal as well as a social, interpersonal, dimension. It is suggestive of the idea that learned behaviour may play a part in the genesis of criminality in general and possibly in the genesis of sexual offending in a similar way. This micro-social level of explanation appears to link behaviour experienced, under defined circumstances, to individuals' future behaviour, health or patterns of cognitive mental structuring. In other words, social and psychological experiences appear to have consequences for future social and psychological behaviour.

In current clinical psychotherapy work at HMP Grendon with sexual offenders a noticeable co-existence of sexual abuse is found together with sexual offending in the life histories of those convicted of sexual offences, in what appears to be a consistently recurring pattern. Some who have experienced sexual abuse do not go on to offend sexually,[3,4] others may develop psychological distress or illness[5] and yet others enter a violent criminal career. Some do not go on to offend at all. There is no absolutely clear pattern[6] found in Widom and Ames's research sample, but a greater link between childhood sexual abuse and later perpetration of violence than of sexual offending was found than directly with sexual abuse. In a non-forensic and perhaps atypical college student sample, childhood sexual abuse was not as likely to lead to later psychological damage or criminal outcome as has sometimes been argued.[7] A UK study concluded 'we do not know' what connection there is between childhood sexual abuse and later sexual offending as the evidence for such a link was inconclusive.[8]

There is, if the evidence is examined closely, a consistently higher clustering of sexually abusive experience in the sexual offender group's earlier life history. These experiences tend to be of longer duration; are often accompanied by greater violence and use of emotional or physical force and are found in the absence of alternative attachments which might ameliorate the destructive effects of undiluted exposure to abusive sexual experience. These apparently linked, co-occurring phenomena, while not representing a causally watertight argument, one phenomenon clearly causing the other, do not appear easy to explain away as unconnected to an offending career in some form. The question remains, what kind of connection is there and what creates the linkage between sexual abuse and sexual offending?

Since 1995, men entering the five therapeutic communities at Grendon have been routinely interviewed on arrival and asked at initial psychological screening whether they have been subject to violence, sexual or other abuses. The figures from the Grendon research department's database between 1995–2002 show that of those who have committed violent offences, 40% reported experience of childhood sexual abuse and of those who had committed sexual offences, 60% reported experience of childhood sexual abuse. In a self-report study in the USA of 301 incarcerated adult male felons of all offence types, 26% of sexual offenders reported childhood sexual abuse and 13% of violent offenders reported childhood sexual abuse.[9]

Not all who have been sexually abused go on to sexually abuse others in the Grendon sample alone. However, while there is an absence of a strong causal link between the two phenomena, there remains something phenomenologically unsatisfying about the absence of a clear enough explanation for the apparent and significant difference in the rates of sexual abuse and sexual offending, particularly when compared with the rates of sexual abuse and sexual offending found in general population studies or in contrast with other offender groups such as violent offenders.

In a UK general population questionnaire survey to family doctors, police surgeons, paediatricians and child psychiatrists, 1 in 6000 children in a year or 3 in 1000 over the whole course of childhood were found to have been sexually abused as children.[10] In a major meta-analytic survey of sexual abuse in the general population, including non-contact abuse, 12% of females and 8% of males reported sexual abuse in childhood, a figure very considerably lower than the rate found in the Grendon database.[11] Consistency in the co-occurrence of clearly higher rates of sexual abuse in the sexual offender population, at least at Grendon, appears to recur across time and require explanation.

Much of the data on sexual abuse is taken from retrospective studies and these have been criticised as unreliable due to: the possibility of subjects responding in a socially desirable manner; the effects of amnesia affecting subjects' recall;[12] and simple misrepresentation for a variety of motives such as hoping for more sympathetic treatment or for improved parole prospects. A number of studies have considered this question and the findings are varied. Some find young men particularly prone to misrepresenting their experiences of abuse if asked about it, because of the need to avoid being thought homosexual.[13] Another approach from the quantitative research field has been to view retrospectively gathered data as questionable because it cannot be objectively verified. While undoubtedly valid, these objections potentially put to one side a wealth of data: men's life stories that might be capable of illuminating the subject of meaning in the field of sexual abuse and sexual offending.

The reliability of retrospective interview research data

More recently qualitative researchers have found ways of cross-checking data so that it can be regarded as more reliable. After many years of research attempting to examine the cycle of abuse theory, Cathy Widom concluded in a later publication[14] that retrospective data on the subject of sexual abuse is not only generally reliable but that interviewees tend to under-report abuse due to the painful and often traumatic effect of these abuses. It was found in the sample of court-substantiated cases of sexual abuse that during research interviews many years later, even though it was known from objective medical and legal sources that sexual abuse had taken place, a number of their subjects did not or could not recall their abuse. Other authors argue that under-reporting of sexual abuse is substantial, particularly among women victims, but evidence is gathering that among men the same under-reporting effect can be found.[3,15] A way through these uncertainties appears in the use of multiple methods within the same study in researching the difficult subject of abuse. Cross-checking official data sources by using triangulation methods[16] such as comparing retrospective interview data with court, psychology and probation reports, police evidence, victim statements and trial judge's summaries may help offer a higher degree of overall objectivity in studies primarily reliant for new data on self-reporting of experiences which may have happened long ago.

The Grendon research project on sexual abuse and sexual offending

A research project, part of a Masters Degree thesis, was carried out for the University of Cambridge Department of Criminology at HMP Grendon on the subject of sexual abuse and sexual offending. It was thought that the personally distant nature of quantitative research might not easily enable it as a method to access meaning or motive in sexual offending. In the field of epistemology problems appear in the application of some social research methodology.[17,18] Specifically that the more distant, non-contact questionnaire forms of quantitative research consistently uncover lower rates of sexual abuse than do the personal, in-depth interview styles of qualitative research. What is happening here? Are there flaws in the quantitative method that hinder the accuracy of what can be understood as social facts in depth derived from research in this field? There seem to be specific factors in research methods that help or hinder access to critically important social facts, such as how many men have been sexually abused and in what kind of way. Access to these social facts is difficult in a subject so fraught with embarrassment, anger, shame and fear. In order to try to overcome some of these methodological problems the philosophical approach adopted in this research project was phenomenological, and an in-depth focus on each man's experience of his abuses, as well as a picture of his whole life's experience, was identified as the field of study. This is to be examined for meaning and any possible link between his sexual offending and his own personal experience of sexual abuse.

The research setting

HMP Grendon is a male category 'B' high security prison run as a series of five therapeutic communities and one induction and assessment unit for men with sentences longer than four years. Men admitted have expressed a wish to engage in therapy and change their offending behaviour and lifestyle. Twelve men convicted of sexual crimes who had also made it known that they had been sexually abused were selected for the research on a 'first come, first served' basis after a request was put to the five communities for volunteers to make themselves known to the researcher. These 12 were given a semi-structured interview which included 24 neutral questions about friends, family, work, school and good experiences and 25 questions about specific and detailed aspects of their sexual life and experiences, including sexual abuses. Permission was obtained from all interviewees, who signed a 'permission to be interviewed' form prior to commencing the research, which specified that their confidentiality would be guaranteed. The project was described to them as an enquiry into the life histories of those who had both offended sexually and been subject to sexual abuse. Only those who had both offended sexually and been subjected to sexual abuse themselves were selected for interview, with the aim of focusing more sharply on what might link these two phenomena. The sample was, therefore, small and highly selective and was an exploratory study into the area of the possible meaning of sexual offending. Any findings, therefore, are of a suggestive nature, requiring further future research to confirm.

Interviews were open-ended, were carried out by the author, who had been trained as a psychotherapist, and took as much time as each man felt he needed to tell his own story. The author attempted to develop a good rapport with each interviewee, taking time to explain the purpose of the research and in the knowledge that it was unlikely that sensitive accounts of experiences of abuse would be made by interviewees unless they felt they could trust the author and could identify the research aim as having real relevance to their lives.

Interviews remained focused so that every man answered exactly the same series of questions but in varying time frames. A triangulation of methods was used and in the first part (1) a pilot study was carried out on six sexual offenders to find out what kinds of abuses they may have experienced and whether they had been sexually abused as well as having committed sexual offences. The six were known to the author but records only were used to establish facts. It was found that of the six sampled, five had both committed sexual offences and also been sexually abused. All six of the sample had experienced more than one kind of abuse, broadly categorised as: violent; sexual; emotional and neglectful abuse. In the second part (2) 12 men were interviewed in depth and their narratives examined for details of the four kinds of abuses noted, together with further detail about the kinds of sexual abuses they had experienced. It was already known that all 12 had committed sexual offences. Detail was sought at interview about what kinds of abuses had been experienced and what effect emotionally and cognitively these experiences had made on each interviewee. Lastly (3) permission was sought for interviewees' records to be checked in order to contrast their life stories with known official records. In part three, two men had left Grendon and one man died before this part of the research had been completed. Nine men's records were examined and included in this part of the research.

In order to give consistency to the research project, definitions were used to judge the presence or absence of the four abuses set as the independent variables against which the histories of offending behaviour and personal abuse were subsequently evaluated. The definitions used to code the presence of the four abuses are taken from the work of Bifulco, Brown and Harris,[19] and Weeks and Widom.[9]

Definitions for neglectful, violent, emotional and sexual abuses

Sexual abuse was defined as present if the sexual act was (1) unwanted, (2) perpetrated by someone five years or more older than the victim, (3) defined as abusive by the interviewee.

Violent abuse was included if (1) independent witnesses could have recorded bruising or marks of beating, (2) hard objects or fists were used, (3) violence occurred frequently and was not an isolated, atypical incident.

Neglectful abuse was present if (1) the interviewee reported being so hungry that he had to go outside the home to search for food or (2) he was given to other carers for significant periods of more than one month at a time and the primary care-giver appeared to have clearly withdrawn from meaningful contact with the interviewee for similar periods at a time.

Emotional abuse was present if (1) anger and belittling, (2) blame or (3) ignoring the interviewee was a dominant attribute of their experienced attachment behaviour, and if it occurred more frequently in the subject than with other siblings.

Findings from the Grendon research

Key research findings from the interviews were that 10 (83%) of the 12 had experienced sexualisation of care-giving relationships involving penetrative sex or masturbation to orgasm by key care-givers. Nine (75%) of the twelve defined home as an unsafe place, giving examples of violent, emotional or sexually abusive behaviour that led to their preferring to be out playing, away at relatives or friends' houses or away from the home in some clear way. More specifically focusing on the commission of the offences of each man, seven of the twelve (58%) demonstrated a recapitulation of the original abuse scenario in the index offence pattern. Recapitulation meant that there were similarities on three levels of comparability between the details of personal abuse suffered and the details of the offence committed. This is not an exact recapitulation but a strikingly similar coincidence of detail outlined in the narrative sequences described below. There was a clear presence, acknowledged by the offender at interview, of specific revenge fantasies associated with earlier abusive experiences and anger, humiliation and rage derived from these abuses, fuelling the commission of the index offence in 10 (83%) of the 12 men interviewed and described by them as clearly present in their thinking before and during the commission of their offences.

These four dominant psycho-social themes emerging from the research have been coded and grouped after McAdams,[20] McAdams and de St Aubin[21] and Maruna,[22] who describe life stories as important and legitimate psycho-social windows into self-concept and possibly motivation. The definitions used to define then code these emergent themes found in the data are described on the page opposite.

Definitions for the four emergent themes

Home was defined as an unsafe place if the interviewee stated it was not safe in response to a direct question, with accompanying narrative evidence indicating why it was unsafe due to violent, sexually abusive or emotionally abusive behaviour from parents or care-givers.

Sexualisation of care-giving relationships was judged present if parents or substitute parents engaged in penetrative or masturbatory sexual activity to orgasm with a boy 'in trust', reported in the narrative or officially documented but not mentioned at interview (one case).

Revenge fantasies were judged present if a strong wish for retribution or revenge was expressed in the interview towards the victim. These appeared fuelled by angry recall of personal abuses and humiliating scenarios and appeared triggered by the behaviour of the victim, cognitively misconstrued by the offender into a rejecting, humiliating scenario which gave reason for attack.

Recapitulation of the original abusive experience in the index offence was judged present if the crime and personal experience of sexual abuse had (1) the setting in which the abuse was committed, (2) the detail of both acts and (3) an expressed intention to repeat what had been done to the interviewee in common.

The kinds of sexual abuses experienced by the interviewees were all of a severe kind, being forced or violent. The qualitative nature of their experiences mainly featured an absence of mutuality, affection or reciprocity between the abuser and abused that might usually be expected to accompany normal sexual relationships. The sexual act had become a breach of trust and a misuse of the power relationship between the younger victim and older abuser. In either learning theory or attachment theory the effect produced appeared likely to be contaminating of good, secure attachment or relationship styles. A selection of sequences from the interview narratives outlined below illustrates the emotional impact of these abusive acts. Typically there was confusion expressed, as some occurrences of sexual abuse could be enjoyable when accompanied by treats – in one case, trips to Burger King, or when some of the relating style of the abuser was affectionate or friendly. Older women abusers were more often viewed as not really abusive (two cases). Examining the narratives closely, it was evident in most cases that the perceived good aspects of sexual abuse tended to occur in the absence of any other good attachment at that time and arguably might not have taken place had there been good attachments available instead of abusive ones. Just six interviewees' narrative accounts have been selected for reasons of economy of space and for the particular narrative clarity of these men's stories. The numbering of the selected quotes, one to six, applies to the six selected throughout the three sets of quotes outlined in Tables 9.1 to 9.3.

Table 9.1 Sexual abuse sequences from the interview narratives

1 Between 12 and 13 there was full sexual intercourse with mother. When she rejected him after this abuse, two older male care staff both anally raped him on Christmas Eve on being received into care: '. . . they drove me off up to this children's home, Beaton Loft, that's where he (the head of home) sodomised me.'

2 Sexual abuse was petting in bed with an older woman at the age of eight. Undisclosed at interview, but confirmed in official probation records was penetrative sexual abuse by male care-workers when in care. Later the interviewee frequented public toilets and engaged in frequent masturbation of older men for money from age nine onwards.

3 At eight he was raped by an older man once, then sexually abused by an uncle by anal intercourse and masturbation for a further five years. 'Things just got more and more, until we ended up in bed, with him laying on top of me and putting himself inside me.'

4 'I went to the class one day . . . I was bleeding and I had sores on my bottom and when I sat down, I basically passed out with pain . . . I'd just been raped.' After being tied up, sometimes blindfolded and anally raped, then left for hours tied up at a time continually between ages 15 and 22, 'There's part of a knuckle missing where I used a razor blade that I hid in my shoes to try and cut myself free.'

5 Oral sex and masturbation took place with brother's friend age seven. Local vicar, age nine '. . . caught me stealing and (said) if you don't do as I say I'll tell your dad and you know what will happen then . . . that was degrading that'. Anal sexual abuse and penetration with candles took place one year and 'I think it was the pain if I'm honest with you that stopped me (going back to him). I used to go home with my fucking, you know, underpants full of blood . . .'

6 'When you're flung over a bed and your pants are ripped off and the man sticks it in your arse, basically, yeah, that's violent. That's what I'm trying to put across to you, that's how it started you see.'

All of the sexually abusive experiences described above were not disclosed to parents and were suffered by the interviewees on their own, except in one case, when the boy disclosed to an 'uncle' who then chased away the abuser and took on the role of abuser in turn himself. Reasons for non-disclosure were not specifically sought but anecdotally included fear and shame. Some of the experiences are clearly violent and were reported as such. As none of the abuses related in the narratives were reported to anyone it might be wondered where the impact of such profound and emotionally affecting experience could go: how did the boys, as they then were, cope? Some of the narrative accounts indicate thinking and emotional reactions welling up often a long way into the future for the interviewees and for some these violent and angry thoughts and feelings became vengeful and appeared in part to take the form of attacks on their victims. Two accounts made clear that it was not important who the victim was but only that someone was going to be targeted as a victim.

Does the concept of recapitulation or of offence-paralleling experience give expression to a proportion of trauma or damage done by abusive experience or is any similarity found merely coincidental? Again, sequences from the interview narratives below illustrate what could appear as recapitulations of original abuse within the index offence pattern. These are inevitably selective, but illustrate the kind of repetition referred to, never exact, but sufficiently similar to raise the heuristic question: are these meaningful links of an identifiable kind between past experience and present behaviour?

Table 9.2 Recapitulation of original abuse within index offence pattern

Interviewee	Recapitulation of sexual abuse within index offence pattern
1	Sexual abuse was a sexual relationship with mother age 12 to 13 then aged 13 anal rape by two older male staff in a children's home. *Crime was the kidnap, violent assault and rape of an elderly woman.* 'I came to do it through fantasising for a lot of years, sleeping with my mother again, wanting to sleep with my mother again, and fantasising (sexually) about older women all the time.'
2	Sexual abuse was sexual initiation by an older woman age eight then sexual abuse by male care-workers (undisclosed at interview but reported in probation reports). *Crime was the rape and false imprisonment of two prostitutes.* 'It was the only time in my life that I ever felt in control of anything, was when I offended.'
3	Original sexual abuse was rape by one man at eight then systematic penetrative abuse till 13 by an uncle. Stepfather very violent: he murdered a woman stranger. *Crime was rape, assault and murder: tied victim to railway lines.* 'She hit me because she realised what I wanted to do . . . I just lost my temper, punched and kicked her, exactly the same way I used to be punched and kicked when I was little.'
4	Sexual abuse was tying up and hooding from age nine and from 15; tying up, hooding and anal sexual assault by an older male relative. *Crime was false imprisonment and indecent assault (tying up a willing paid volunteer and attempting masturbation).* 'I knew being abused was wrong, I knew being raped was wrong, I knew having something in your sphincter was wrong, but when it got to tying up, the original bit, I didn't really relate that to being wrong.'
5	Original sexual abuse was sexual intercourse with an older boy and rape and sexual assault by a vicar for one year age nine. *Crime was the rape and violent assault of a young boy who allegedly looked like the interviewee.* 'David looked like me and I suppose I subjected David to the same stuff Bruce subjected me to. And for years before the offence I was carrying all this stuff, I was carrying a lot of anger, a lot of hatred, and I wanted other people to suffer, and now it was my turn to be in control.'
6	Original sexual abuse was fondling then anal rape over one year by an older man, a publican. *Crime was the indecent assault and wounding of a woman.* 'But the day I created the victims . . . that's when I ceased becoming a victim myself.'

The impact of these abuses appears clearly enough in the men's accounts and was not difficult to associate in the men's thinking with the offences they had committed. What effect do such abuses have on the men's sense of self? The interview narratives were dominated by negative or contaminating sequences which were judged likely to hinder each man's generative potential to lead a life regularly attuned to the feelings and needs of others. This was found despite the deliberate series of questions included which had aimed to elicit any good, redeeming experiences.

Table 9.3 Self-concept sequences

Interviewee	Self-concept sequences
1	'Tired . . . I guess the most honest one of the lot would be struggling . . . swimming against what seems a tide.'
2	'I used to feel disgusted with myself.'
3	'I always see myself as an underachiever like and I might go so far as to say worthless piece of shit, but there you go.'
4	'I have basically been the person that's basically had the family to stay together, do what they wanted to do and as a result of everybody else's pleasure. I've been that piece of meat.'
5	'I didn't think anything of myself. I don't think I've ever really achieved anything in life.'
6	'I've never self-harmed, I don't believe in cutting myself up, I was too busy doing it the other way round . . . through the football, that's were I was getting my release, I was taking anger out.'

Discussion of the findings

The six narrative sequences selected above have been chosen to illustrate the powerful impact of the interviewees' sexually abusive experience on them. The six life story accounts excluded contain similar examples but those selected have been chosen for their narrative clarity. The impact of sexually abusive experience seems to be equated with something similar to an act of violence, particularly when the interviewee felt unable to object to what was taking place. A reaction of anger associated with feelings of revenge appears to accompany acts of sexual violation in the narratives, although most of the interviewees had experienced more than one of the four abuses identified in the research. This complicates the research picture. A most striking aspect of the abusive scenario remains the assumption of powerlessness to alter the course of abuse made by the interviewees who in all 12 cases felt unable to act to defend themselves. All but one never spoke about it to anyone for months or years. One man had told no one about his experiences for 40 years and only did so because he was in therapy.

It emerged as critical to this study to have used the style of an exploratory psychotherapeutic interview in combination with the precision of a tight interview schedule of questions asked of all subjects. It was clearly important to take care to develop a good rapport with the interviewees, what might be thought of as a temporary working relationship, and it seemed unlikely that the same kind of narrative detail would have been forthcoming from the interviews without such care and attention.

The impression gained from this small, exploratory study sample is of a group who have mostly experienced multiple abuses which have taken place over a long period of time and in which abuse has been exclusively forced (non-consensual) and traumatic. Anal rape took place in eight cases and forced oral sex with an older man in two further cases. When sexual abuses are set within the context of a multiple abuse attachment configuration, including neglect, abandonment, violent or emotional abuse, then the likelihood of victims taking up perpetrator status appears further strengthened in this sample. This strengthening appears to be associated with the predominance of contaminating over redeeming attachment experience and the possibility that such a disproportionate weighting of negative over positive experience has psychological consequences in later life. There is a strong argument that these abusive experiences shape the quality of the internal working models of relationship life that later become the men's learned behavioural repertoire.

This study's finding that ten of the interviewees (83%) had experienced sexualisation of key care-giving relationships accords with Watkins and Bentovim's[23] extensive review of research on sexual abuse, in which they conclude that factors making a perpetrator outcome more likely in those that have been sexually abused are '. . . a combination of sexualisation and externalising responses'. If there is any direction that research might take in the future, it would seem to need to be in discovering more about the personal life experience of those who have offended sexually and those who have been subjected to sexual abuses in careful in-depth interview studies.

In this sample, sexual assault appears as a violent expression of attachment and discharge-seeking behaviour, as the interviewees' narratives indicate, with considerable hatred and unhappiness wedded to the sexual act itself. It is no longer an enjoyable act but an act more akin to revenge or retaliation. Describing sexual perversion as an 'erotic form of hatred', Stoller[24] points to the occurrence of a discharge of such powerful feelings as hatred and rage in the sexual act of perversion. Hatred and sex become fused in a joint action, a repetition, which appears to give expression to powerful internally held trauma, evident in the narrative accounts given in this study.

The psychoanalytic repetition compulsion and what is more recently described in cognitive psychology as 'offence-paralleling behaviour'[25] address this tendency to enact and repeat offending behaviour. The point is the same, that offending behaviour seems to repeat itself over time. What is different between the theories is that psychoanalytic theory holds that behaviour tends not only to be learned and repeated but has specific unconscious meaning that may not be understood until carefully worked through into consciousness through the process of therapy, or until the behaviour no longer functions to give symptomatic relief. Psychoanalytic thinking also holds that there is a relationship between past experience and present behaviour and that when the loading of pathology is great enough, or when there are a sufficient number of negative attachment associations located in the sexual act, then it is likely to be the sexual act through which that pathology becomes acted out: the offence itself. The act of sexual attack appears to take on an outward form of expression of what has been perversely experienced and incorporated internally by the offender, at least in part, and which he appears to need to rid himself of through the activity of offending: acting out.

The psychotherapeutic intention at Grendon is that new non-perverse relationship and behavioural models are intentionally made available over time in therapy and through the example and modelling of staff, and of inmates who are sufficiently able to act as pro-social models. These serve to replace the original violent, abusive and perverse models and these new models are eventually understood and incorporated as a new part of the offender's behavioural repertoire. Not all are amenable to changing their behaviour at Grendon, but many are. These new models hopefully function to redress the offending impulse and the apparent tendency to re-enact and repeat abuses, often in an escalating and worsening pattern, that have been perpetrated often long ago.

Quotes used in the narrative themes cited in this study have been reproduced with the interviewees' written permission to do so.

References

1 Padfield N (2000) *Criminal Law* (2e). Butterworths, London.
2 Fattah EA (ed.) (1992) *Towards a Critical Victimology*. St Martin's Press, New York and Basingstoke.
3 Finkelhor D (1984) *Child Sexual Abuse: new theory and research*. Free Press, New York.
4 West DJ, Roy C and Nichols FL (1978) *Understanding Sexual Attacks*. Heinemann Educational Books Limited, London.
5 Finkelhor D (1990) Early and long-term effects of child sexual abuse: an update. *Professional Psychology: Research and Practice*. **21**: 325–30.
6 Widom CS and Ames MA (1994) Criminal consequences of childhood sexual victimization. *Child Abuse and Neglect*. **18**: 303–18.
7 Rind B, Tromovich P and Bauserman R (1998) A meta-analytic examination of assumed properties of childhood sexual abuse using college samples. *Psychological Bulletin*. **124**(1): 22–53.
8 Grubin D (2001) *Sex Offending Against Children: understanding the risk*. Home Office Research, Development and Statistics Directorate. Police Research Series, Paper 99.
9 Weeks R and Widom CS (1998) Self-reports of early childhood victimization among incarcerated adult male felons. *Journal of Interpersonal Violence*. **13**(3): 346–61.
10 Mrazek PJ, Lynch MA and Bentovim A (1983) Sexual abuse of children in the United Kingdom. *Child Abuse and Neglect*. **7**: 147–53.
11 Baker AW and Duncan SP (1985) Child sexual abuse: a study of prevalence in Great Britain. *Child Abuse and Neglect*. **9**: 457–64.
12 Briere J (1992) Methodological issues in the study of sexual abuse effects. *Journal of Consulting and Clinical Psychology*. **60**: 196–203.
13 Freeman-Longo RE (1986) The impact of sexual victimization on males. *Child Abuse and Neglect*. **10**: 411–14.
14 Widom CS and Morris S (1997) Accuracy of adult recollections of childhood victimization: Part 11: Childhood sexual abuse. *Psychological Assessment*. **9**(1): 34–46.
15 Scott S (2001) *Out of the Shadows: help for men who have been sexually assaulted*. Russell House Press, Lyme Regis.
16 Bachman R and Schutt RK (2001) *The Practice of Research in Criminology and Criminal Justice*. Sage, Thousand Oaks, CA.
17 Goldman JDG and Padayachi UK (2000) Some methodological problems in estimating incidence and prevalence in child sexual abuse research. *The Journal of Sex Research*. **37**(4): 305–14.

18 Consiorek JC, Bera WH and LeTourneau D (1994) *Male Sexual Abuse: a trilogy of intervention strategies.* Sage, Thousand Oaks, CA.

19 Bifulco A, Brown GW and Harris TO (1994) Childhood Experience of Care and Abuse (CECA): a retrospective interview measure. *Journal of Child Psychology and Psychiatry.* 35(8): 1419–35.

20 McAdams DP (1993) *The Stories We Live By: personal myths and the making of the self.* Morrow, New York.

21 McAdams DP and de St Aubin E (1992) A theory of generativity and its assessment through self-reports, behavioural acts, and narrative themes in autobiography. *Journal of Personality and Social Psychology.* 62: 1003–15.

22 Maruna S (2001) *Making Good: how ex-convicts reform and rebuild their lives.* American Psychological Association, Washington, DC.

23 Watkins WGA and Bentovim A (1992) The sexual abuse of male children and adolescents: a review of current research. *Journal of Child Psychology and Psychiatry.* 33(1): 197–248.

24 Stoller RJ (1975, reprinted 1986) *Perversion: the erotic form of hatred.* Quartet Books, London.

25 Cullen E, Jones L and Woodward R (1997) *Therapeutic Communities for Offenders.* John Wiley & Sons, Chichester.

Chapter 10

Murder as an attempt to manage self-disgust

David Jones

One man smashes the skull of a friend, cuts off his penis and drowns him in apparent response to a crude remark about his sexuality. A second turns to see an acquaintance undoing the trousers of a friend and commits a murder of quite extreme proportions, again involving mutilation of the victim's penis. The third kills in fear of having his homosexuality exposed, not least to himself, and later comes to believe that he was the victim of a conspiracy. In each of these cases the perpetrator claimed to be disgusted and outraged at the actions of the victim.

This chapter looks at disgust and the way that murder sometimes represents the extreme end of a range of responses to the feeling of disgust. I have observed aspects of this dynamic most clearly in relation to homosexuality or more precisely to a fear of homosexuality, and the chapter does focus upon this area. However, I am not claiming that this is exclusively so nor indeed that homosexuality necessarily evokes feelings of disgust. Indeed, since I am suggesting that the response arises from the externalisation of an internal dynamic I would speculate that this feature also contributes to the causation of a number of other violent sexual acts, for example child killing following a sexual attack. A simple example occurs towards the beginning of Stephen King's novel *Carrie*. Following a near riot in the girl's showers the Gym teacher, Miss Desjardin, had her white shorts smeared with Carrie's menstrual blood: '[her] face contorted into a pucker of disgust, and she suddenly hurled Carrie, stumbling, to her feet.' Later she confessed: 'I understand how those girls felt. The whole thing made me want to take the girl and shake her'.[1] Furthermore, I am quite clear that this is a different phenomenon from the highly sadistic psychopathology associated with such serial murderers as Jeffrey Dahmer or John Wayne Gacy. Many attempts are made to forge a connection between these examples and homosexuality in general, particularly by the religious right wing in the USA, and they are often in the guise of scientific papers.[2] These attempts are frequently facile and serve only to restrict thought around the area. Indeed, they may represent a different presentation of the phenomenon under discussion in this chapter. However, there is no doubt that there are a large number of men in our prisons who have committed murder following some sexual contact with another man and it is the nature of this complex and strongly ambivalent sequence of feelings and actions that I explore.

This dynamic also has some importance to us in the psychological professions in terms of transference and countertransference interactions, in other words how we feel and how we respond to our clients. This can arise because of a widespread unease about polymorphous sexuality and the phenomenon of universal bisexuality producing self-disgust. Because this discomfort is usually denied or unconscious it cannot be eliminated through the simple imposition of rules or protocols, although these can have some value in maintaining reasonable standards of social behaviour, at work, for example. However, it is crucial to be aware of this possibility or work with clients can be compromised.[3]

Disgust, shame and aggression

Disgust

The affect of disgust has been relatively little examined in the literature and yet it is very common in everyday life. Susan Miller attributes this to the fear of contamination that is central to disgust reactions. Contact with the disgusting makes one disgusting.[4] A friend of mine recently gave me a simple example of the ease of transmission of disgust. He was enjoying a prawn cocktail on the patio of a restaurant when he was approached by a beautiful cat. As the cat turned round it displayed a wide area of its face with the skin torn back exposing the flesh. He was filled with disgust and since then has not been able to even think of a prawn cocktail without a feeling of nausea.

For Darwin, the term 'disgust' meant something offensive to taste. He thought that it primarily arose in connection with eating or tasting, thus the emotion causes characteristic movements of the mouth and face. But it also often provokes annoyance in the subject, hence a frown is a frequent feature. Extreme disgust makes the subject look as if he is about to vomit. Retching or vomiting may be induced by a thought, particularly if it is associated with some previously disgusting object, as an impression may be retained and transferred to other similar objects. Smell is also a powerful evoker.[5]

Freud identified disgust, shame and morality as the forces which acted against sexual development, seeing them as arising from inhibitory factors, externally applied in the long process of the emotional development of the human race.[6]

A helpful perspective on disgust was offered by Shand[7] from outside the field of psychology. At its primitive level disgust is a physical impulse rather than an emotion; indeed, when the physical sensations are strongest they tend to dominate the attention and emotion will be absent. This impulse is concerned with forcefully ejecting something from the body or withdrawing from something that repulses. The *emotion* of disgust will only develop, or perhaps be exposed, when the bodily sensations are not so intense as to absorb attention. The emotion causes us to turn away from its object. A crucial observation contributed in this philosophical study is that disgust tends to repress pity so we are more likely to feel contempt for the disgusting object.

To summarise, disgust is an affect probably originally founded in response to bad tastes and smells with their link to spoiled food and over the ages generalised to certain tactile experiences, sliminess for example, and further extended to thoughts of something expected to be disgusting. The development of disgust seems to be culturally related, is easily transferred and now includes not just threat to the body but threat to the soul or core self.[8] Furthermore, it features in interpersonal relationships, where it is experienced as a response to others. Characteristically it entails a powerful emotional or physical rejection of someone felt to be threatening an invasion of the self. It may be expressed through rejection, attacking or nauseated tolerance.[4] The disgusting object is believed to be tainted, damaged and irreparable.

My suggestion in this chapter is that for some people the disgust is directed towards a part of themselves and that the power of the experience is such as to provoke extreme fear and panic. The internal integrity is so threatened as to demand immediate evacuation, to emotionally vomit. The disgusting part may then be split off and projected onto some other person or some other part of the self. Aggression may thus also be directed outwards and thereby some temporary relief is gained from perpetual self denigration and depression but to the cost of intimacy in personal relationships, emotional impoverishment and in extreme cases an attempt to destroy the contaminated object.

Shame

Unlike disgust, shame has received a great deal of attention over the past 30 years or so. While it was initially regarded as an internal barrier to the libido,[9] a broader definition seems to be emerging. Central to this is the feeling of being exposed, of one's failure being on view to some other. The circularity of this increases a 'tormenting sense of inferiority and sinfulness'.[10] It arises from exposure that threatens the integrity of the self, 'or the self defined as a self before others'.[11] A number of writers have also identified a connection between the avoidance of shame and aggression.[11,12,13] Thomas argues that shame is a primitive physiological response to a rejection of oneself by another. It may be experienced as an intense pain which stimulates anger and violence which in turn may be directed outwards toward another or inward against oneself.[14,11]

Thus shame can be seen as a complex emotion, linked to the superego, or critical conscience, and operating as a dynamic inhibiting the impulses of the id through the production of emotional pain. If the perceived failing is split off and projected outwards it can produce disgust towards the object which is the recipient or, if split off and internalised, it may act as the focus for disgust with self. If the pain is strong it may produce anger and aggression which, according to the status of the projections, may be directed towards self or others.

The notion of the internal world

The idea that a part of the mind may set itself against another part of itself or may split itself off and be located with another person or object is by no means straightforward particularly when mentioned at the same time as the unconscious to which it is closely allied. Empirically based psychologists have long denied the existence of an unconscious preferring to consider behaviours which can be observed, measured, calibrated and manipulated. However, psychotherapists, particularly psychoanalytic psychotherapists, also observe. They observe the behaviour of clients during therapy sessions, the nuances and changes of feeling, the presentation of material and the effect that this has upon them and they infer a meaning from this to bring into focus the status of the client's internal world.

More recently there has been a degree of rapprochement between these two wings of the field of psychology. Empirical psychologists have been able to devise experiments which demonstrate the existence of an unconscious and such phenomena as transference.[15] The development of cognitive behavioural approaches recognises the importance of feelings as well as behaviours, and schema theories[16] illustrate the existence of structures of belief below the level of conscious thinking. Still, these seem to be describing essentially static scripts which cause particular behaviours and this is very different from the idea of a dynamic internal world where elements of the personality are in perpetual interaction with other elements and with the outside world. The psychoanalyst Melanie Klein described it thus:

> 'The baby, having incorporated his parents feels them to be live people inside his body in the concrete way in which deep unconscious phantasies are experienced . . . They are in his mind, "internal" or "inner" objects, as I have termed them. Thus an inner world is being built up in the child's unconscious mind, corresponding to his actual experiences and the impressions he gains from people and the external world and yet altered by his own phantasies and impulses. If it is a world of people predominantly at peace with each other and with the ego, inner harmony, security, and integration ensue.'[17]

As Klein suggests, the internal world is affected both by internal relations and the impact of the external world and the degree of personality well-being and integration is dependent upon these internal relations. A psychological defence that splits off a disagreeable or unacceptable part of the personality and locates it in the external world or even an area of the internal world that is experienced as being separate from the central ego can bring some relief but only at the price of a fresh discord or general impoverishment of the personality. When this splitting occurs then the critical object which may give rise to feelings of inadequacy, shame or disgust can appear to become more persecutory and so set off a cycle of violence which leads to murder or suicide.[18]

Homosexuality, disgust and bisexuality

Over time homosexuality has been regarded as a sin, a crime and an illness,[19] and while the term homosexuality itself was coined as recently as 1869 by Karoly Maria Kertbeny, there has been unease throughout history and in parts of the world and within certain cultures the unease is as strong as ever. Witness the declaration by Pope John Paul II, who described same-sex relationships as evil and continued:

> 'This judgement does not permit us to conclude that all those who suffer from this anomaly are personally responsible for it but it does attest to the fact that homosexual acts are intrinsically disordered.'[20]

During the first half of the twentieth century German fascists regarded homosexuals as degenerates fit for eradication. As Himmler said, '[drowning in a swamp] was not a punishment, but simply the extinguishing of abnormal life. It had to be got rid of, just as we pull out the weeds, throw them on a heap and burn them.'[21] Schools of thought developed within psychology that homosexuals needed changing, indeed should be changed.[3,22] So throughout the institutions of human society the great passions of shame, anger and disgust have fuelled widespread homophobic attitudes. In effect, same-sex intimacy becomes the receptacle for all that is feared and unwanted and thus despised. In excising the latent homosexuality and locating it elsewhere, social groups take a short cut from the dilemma posed by universal bisexuality and the uncomfortable matter of the Oedipal triangle of child, mother, and father. This often results in rigid and sometimes highly destructive social and legal attitudes.

On an individual level one sees the same pattern repeated. Men who profess the most anti-gay views and the most discomfort with homosexuals show a greater level of sexual arousal on being shown homosexual videos than non-homophobic men.[23] In prisons, a form of paranoia can develop which gives rise to sudden and unexpected violence. James Gilligan uses the term 'homosexual panic'. This occurs when 'an inmate experiences a degree of homosexual stimulation that is intolerable to his self esteem and his sense of his own masculinity'.[24] The confined space and claustrophobic structures of prison can produce such extreme reactions but I would argue that this is only the ordinary individual reaction writ large. For example, a young man, James, described how he had only come to realise that he was gay during his second sexual relationship. When his partner told a third party, James was physically sick. The nausea arose at the point of having to see something about himself that he did not want to see. It was not the content of his stomach that demanded expulsion but a mixture of dread, fear and disgust. Once out, the anxiety diminished and James became accepting of his sexuality.

Two examples of disgust uncovered during psychotherapy

The following two vignettes from individual therapy describe the struggle that two clients, gay men, had accepting their sexuality. These middle class, bright men who appeared to have accepted the fact of their sexual orientation nevertheless experienced strong feelings of self-disgust which had a serious, destructive impact upon their personal relationships.

Philip

Philip is a young man in his early thirties. He came to me because he was feeling depressed. He was infatuated with a friend who had the same name, Phil.

As the therapy continued it became clear that it was important to Philip that he had Phil as the recipient of his positive transference as it allowed him to avoid becoming too intimately involved with me in the therapy.

Phil moved into Philip's house and often his girlfriend would stay overnight. Philip became even more preoccupied by their relationship and would listen with his ear pressed up against the bedroom wall to the sound of their intercourse, waiting for and coveting the sound of the orgasm. Then he would masturbate afterwards. One day he described to me how he had been hanging around downstairs while Phil and girlfriend made love upstairs. He was trapped downstairs and resented missing their orgasm. After they had left for work he went to their room and rummaged for soiled tissues. He liked the smell of the semen and he placed the tissue up his anus imagining that it was Phil's penis but as he did so he said he was disgusted by the thought of the girl's vaginal fluid and this put him off.

He thinks I may be disgusted by it, and that his friend, Phil, would be if he knew. I said to him that the point is that *he, Philip, knows, his thoughts are an indication that a part of him is disgusted.* The masturbation was an attempt to overcome his feeling of isolation and the intense envy of the exclusiveness of the parental couple, but he becomes disgusted at the prurience of his intrusiveness. This was denied and the part of him that was disgusted was projected into me, so reinforcing his experience of a persecuting authority and relieving him of the responsibility of doing anything about it. However, he was also correct in that I did experience strong feelings, particularly about his intrusiveness. The unconscious transference certainly had an erotic element of a masochistic kind to it, being both a statement about his curiosity about me and an attempt to stir up a sadistic response. My response was to feel threatened by the aggressive homosexuality of it. This stopped me responding to the disgust by pointing his intrusiveness out to him, which would have been an appropriate response, but I also experienced some panic, which reduced my capacity to think.

In the event Phil moved away and Philip became steadily more resentful towards me, especially when the girlfriend went to visit Phil. He was stirred up by this, as if this parental couple were getting together behind his back, he felt rejected and marginalised and driven to find some way of acting out the pain and anger by expelling the bad mummy/daddy. Therapy was ended abruptly in a way that both expressed aggressive feelings and avoided the risk of being swamped by feelings of loss or dependency. In effect I had been killed off.

Alan

My second example, Alan, was seen for about six months. He was a man in his late twenties. In the first session he made it clear that he did not want to look at or consider his sexuality. He had, he felt, worked that out for himself and it had been a long and painful process and he did not want it questioned by me. I was one of his 'oppressors', he had decided, therefore I could not understand. Not that he was uncritical of his peers. He once described to me how, at a gay party, he had looked around the room and thought what a useless bunch of depraved freaks he could see. These people disgusted him. He was not objectively describing the people he was with, his friends, peers or colleagues but that he was in the uneasy position of having set himself apart from this group. He despised them or to put it another way he despised a part of himself that had been split off and projected onto others whom it then seemed that he despised.

His presenting problem was that having been in a stable relationship for some seven years he had discovered that he could engage in casual sex and enjoy it. Thus he would frequently visit a public toilet and have sex on his way home from work. This had come to affect his primary relationship and eventually he had told his boyfriend, who was sympathetic and supportive but said that this behaviour would have to stop. He tried but found it difficult and he soon picked up the habit again. It left him feeling depressed and empty.

On one occasion he told me how a police helicopter had been hovering over the public toilets while he was there. He became convinced that it was spying on him to the extent of following him home. In his description of the helicopter he was illustrating just how powerful his mechanisms of splitting and projection were. Through this same process I came to represent the persecuting authority exposing him in all his shame and degradation.

At a point when I felt that we had worked through an issue related to the disappointment and anger he had towards his weak father he terminated the therapy in a sudden and spiteful manner. Arising from material in his dream I had drawn attention to the need to clean up his internal world and indicated to him that I knew that he knew that it was in a disgusting state. He was enraged at that idea and so, like Philip, symbolically killed me off.

These two men experienced a high level of shame. To them the very essence of the analytic work was to uncover the most shameful things and of course this was very threatening. I was the third party pointing a finger and saying 'you are shameful!' More than this, they were disgusted with themselves and despite attempts to locate the disgustingness and its response elsewhere, at both an internal unconscious level and externally, this only provided temporary relief while at the same time spoiling existing relationships.

Those who commit murder

In prison, men are invariably less well integrated, more impulsive, less rooted in a supportive social structure than Philip or Alan. In a high security therapeutic establishment such as Grendon, two-thirds of the men have been without one parent before the age of 16, two-thirds report physical abuse and almost half report sexual abuse. Even allowing for a degree of exaggeration for the purpose of gaining sympathy, such figures are high. Recent court cases relating to offences committed at children's homes over a number of decades have confirmed many of these claims.

A significant number of men are in prison serving life for offences of killing other men following a sexual incident. In such circumstances a common scenario is that the perpetrator knows or is friendly with the victim, may have been drinking or sharing drugs with him and agrees to go with him. He may have sex with the man and kill him afterwards or the murder may be triggered by some related event short of sexual contact.

In the first situation Gary murdered his best friend for making an offensive remark about his sexuality. The murder was out of the blue and the degree of violence extreme. Cutting off the penis represented retribution and revenge, but for what? Although he had a girlfriend at this time he was very uncertain about his sexuality and later became settled in a gay orientation. He had also been sexually abused as a child.

Brian came from an extremely disturbed family. He did not know his father and suffered a series of more or less abusive stepfathers. He was sexually and physically abused as well as being an observer of a sexual assault on his own mother. His murder occurred after he and two friends returned intoxicated to a flat and fell asleep. Brian awoke to find one of them undoing the trousers of the remaining, still asleep, friend. Again, his reaction was notable not just for the violent act but for the extent of the violence. Once control was lost, and Brian is generally a very controlled man, then it was not recovered until the victim had been battered into oblivion and mutilated. There is some evidence that murders involving homosexual victims are more violent than heterosexual victims[25] and this supports the idea that the victim comes to represent some additional quality invested or projected into him by his killer.

In the third situation Malcolm had been developing a relationship with a gay man. Eventually this resulted in a sexual relationship, or so all the evidence indicated. Malcolm feared being blackmailed, that he might be exposed, and this led up to him killing the man and trying to cover his tracks. After several years he discovered a different version of this. This was that he had been kidnapped and subject to violence by a group of men and the killing occurred when he tried to escape. Each of these situations has escape in common. He wanted to escape public labelling as being gay and being labelled gay does have a particularly adhesive quality. Men are outed as gay even if the relationship existed 20 years previously. It never occurs the other way round and it is impossible to lose the label once applied. He wanted to escape the consequences of his actions by hiding his tracks and he wanted to escape self-knowledge by subscribing to an extravagant conspiracy theory. This alteration in his belief, which actually could be most counter-productive to any desire to seek release, needs to be understood as an emotional imperative; he has to find an alternative explanation because the original one is simply unacceptable.

Each of these three men had a deprived and disrupted upbringing set within a culture where drugs and alcohol were easily available. They grew up without firm family boundaries where it was commonplace to slip into petty theft to fund addictive appetites. However, we know that there will be other individuals who emerge from a similar background but who do not follow such a disastrous path. The relevance of this information here is that it helps us to understand something of the fragility of the personality, which is liable to fragment and panic under extreme provocation. What had happened with each of them was that they had been confronted by an internal experience that induced a feeling of extreme anxiety and panic. The panic arose because there seemed to be no escape from the rage and disgust that previously had been repressed, contributing nevertheless to fertile conditions for drug abuse and criminal behaviour. At the breaking point, when the ego structure disintegrates, the victim becomes the recipient of all of these disgusting qualities which are emotionally vomited onto him. At such points the assailant loses all pity for his victim who instead becomes an increasingly critical object as the battering and mutilation progresses. Such a cycle is described by Wilson:[18] 'there is an amplification of violent activity; the object is progressively downgraded and damaged but refuses to lie down, taking on an increasingly persecutory and horrific aspect with each new insult to which it is subjected.'

Working with disgust

The three men described above are all quite pleasant, intelligent men who relate well to others in the bizarre world of a high security prison. They could, however, also be described as callous, lacking empathy or psychopathic. But what would such terms add to our understanding of them and to our ability to help them lead more safe, rewarding and satisfactory lives? Such terms would tell us that they are unemotional, hard to help, manipulative, not to be trusted. All terms that they will be very familiar with since their first case conference at their first children's home. Their most serious crimes were committed in a state of high emotional arousal but allowing access to their emotions is very threatening, very dangerous for them. Most of their lives they have maintained highly developed but dysfunctional defences against these feelings which continually threaten to annihilate them emotionally.

Of course, these defences become rigid, fixed and stereotyped during adulthood, but actually the trick remains the same: to engage them emotionally in a way that allows trust to develop, encourages reflection and permits a renegotiation of the relationship between the core self and the persecuting internal object. Where disgust is concerned this is a very delicate matter since it is such a volatile emotion and the response can be of projectile force. Nevertheless it is important that this area of the inmates' internal world is not overlooked, since it lies dormant until circumstances arise which provoke a reprise.

For the practitioner, working with disgust is difficult and demanding. You can expect your tolerance and experience to be pushed to and beyond the limits. You may feel uncomfortable and worthless but the main danger is responding to these powerful feelings by rejecting or condemning the client.

References

1 King S (1975) *Carrie*. Signet, New York.
2 Cameron P (1993) *Violence and Homosexuality* [Internet article]. www.familyresearchinst.org/FRI_EduPamphlet4.html
3 Jones D (2001) Shame, disgust, anger and revenge: homosexuality and countertransference. *British Journal of Psychotherapy*. **17**(4): 493–504.
4 Miller S (1993) Disgust reactions: their determinants and manifestations in treatment. *Contemporary Psychoanalysis*. **29**(4): 711–35.
5 Darwin C (1965) *The Expression of the Emotions in Man and Animals*. University of Chicago Press, Chicago.
6 Freud S (1905) Three essays on sexuality. Infantile sexuality. In: *On Sexuality*. Pelican Books, London.
7 Shand AF (1914) *The Foundations of Character*. Macmillan, London.
8 Rozin P, Haidt J and McCauley CR (2000) Disgust. In: *Handbook of Emotions* (2e). Guilford Press, New York.
9 Levine S (1971) The psychoanalysis of shame. *International Journal of Psychoanalysis*. **52**(4): 355–62.
10 Berke JH (1986) Shame and envy. *British Journal of Psychotherapy*. **2**(4): 262–70.
11 Lansky MR (1994) Shame: contemporary psychoanalytic perspectives. *Journal of the American Academy of Psychoanalysis*. **22**(3): 433–41.
12 Lansky MR (1991) Shame and the problem of suicide: a family systems perspective. *British Journal of Psychotherapy*. **7**(3): 230–42.
13 Pines M (1995) The universality of shame: a psychoanalytic approach. *British Journal of Psychotherapy*. **11**(3): 346–57.
14 Thomas SE (1995) Experiencing a shame response as a precursor to violence. *Bulletin of the American Academy of Psychiatry Law*. **23**(4): 587–93.
15 Andrews B and Brewin C (2000) What did Freud get right? *The Psychologist*. **13**(10): 605–23.
16 Young JE (1994) *Cognitive Therapy for Personality Disorders: a schema focused approach*. Professional Resources Press, Sarasota, FL.
17 Klein M (1940) Mourning and its relation to manic depressive states. In: *Love, Guilt and Reparation and Other Works*. Hogarth Press, London.
18 Wilson S (1995) *The Cradle of Violence*. Jessica Kingsley, London.
19 Zachary A (2001) Uneasy triangles: a brief overview of the history of homosexuality. *British Journal of Psychotherapy*. **17**(4): 489–92.
20 *Guardian*, 1 August 2003.
21 Burleigh M and Wipperman W (1991) *The Racial State. Germany 1933–1945*. Cambridge University Press, Cambridge.

22 Nicolosi J (1993) *Healing Homosexuality*. Aronson, New Jersey.
23 Adams HE, Wright Jr LW and Lohr B (1996) Is homophobia associated with homosexual arousal? *Journal of Abnormal Psychology*. **105**(3): 440–5.
24 Gilligan J (2000) The symbolism of punishment. In: *Violence: reflections on our deadliest epidemic*. Jessica Kingsley, London.
25 Bell MD and Vila RI (1996) Homicide in homosexual victims. *American Journal of Forensic Medicine and Pathology*. **17**(1): 65–9.

Chapter 11

Working at the coalface

Jane Coltman

When I applied to join the Prison Service I was unsure what to expect in my forthcoming role as a prison officer. After 'five years in' I am starting to realise that this uncertainty about role and ensuing frustrations and challenges are as much a reality of prison work as locks, bars and routine.

Prison staff enforce segregation of prisoners from the outside world. Our key purpose is to keep prisoners in custody. Trainee prison officers, as I found when joining, are weaned onto the ideals of the service, with the doctrine of order and control, at training colleges. Key targets and acronyms become the order of the day. SMART objectives, KPIs (key performance indicators), RE-SPECT and numerous other uncomfortable examples of corporate jargon were learned parrot fashion. By the time it came to learning to march on a parade ground and daily fitness lessons in the gym it became apparent that the Prison Service also emulates the military culture. A high percentage of prison officers are indeed from a military background. No one asked why any of us wanted to become prison officers or what we wished to bring to the role.

Certainly being able to march has never helped me when confronted by an inmate firing verbal abuse, or in tears – sometimes both. Thus we as prison staff seek to impose order and control and containment on those labelled chaotic, disturbed and dangerous. Many prisoners are indeed dangerous. A glance down the roll board in Grendon and many other prisons will confirm this. Over 40% at Grendon are lifers. The remaining 55–60% are recidivist offenders, with sentences of seven years and over – those on a determinate sentence. If these determinates don't reform on the current sentence they will return to prison as two-strike lifers with the knowledge that they have again left more victims. This is an undeniably disturbing fact that cannot be erased from the consciousness of the victims (if alive), the public, law enforcement agencies, policy makers, prison staff, and, too late, by the perpetrator. Regrettably the majority in Britain go on to reoffend. (Have you ever tried significantly changing your own behaviour? Not easy . . .)

The conundrum exists therefore: how do we, as officers, help effect positive change in prisoners, thus reducing risk? Fallible human beings undertaking to reduce risk in the even more disordered! Most would agree prisons are an unnatural environment with protocol, rules and an alien subculture. Yet it is the medium for containing society's and the service's own anxieties about coping with or working with those who have proven their dangerousness and need.

A prisoner entering prison for the first time is at high risk of self-harming or suicide. After this first hurdle he or she is inherently vulnerable to the instant gratification that drug abuse affords. Kicking off, bullying intimidation, dealing, fear and isolation are other coping strategies, for some replicating their lifestyle on the outside, for others experienced when entering the prison system. Add to this poor educational performance, poor social skills, a likely history of parental abuse, and the feeling of being an outsider with little to lose on the outside, and it starts to become clear that change is a complex and controversial task. The majority of these men have committed sickening crimes. Should we punish, control, or first try to gain some understanding of how this catalogue of misery has come into place?

The instinctive response to anything very unpleasant in life is either to react immediately out of panic, or to push the problem away. At the risk of further reducing any small chance of promotion, I would state that the Prison Service also displays these insecurities. These insecurities are of course heightened by (1) political pressure to do something, (2) our innate fear of crime, and (3) a steeply rising prison population.

The more draconian traditional prison traditions – bang-ups, nickings, segregation – are one way of dealing with the problem. Unfortunately, whilst these measures may gain short-term compliance, they replicate the destructive behaviour exhibited by many of the prisoners' parents or the formative influences that have helped place the prisoner on the road of crime, deviance and self-destructiveness in the first place. However, the wider ideals of prison, discipline, enforcing boundaries, challenging selfish and abhorrent behaviour can be seen as a working partnership between therapeutic ideals and the prison system ideals.

Thus at Grendon a multidisciplinary approach exists that aims to gain an understanding of the root causes of the pathology of offending in an attempt to address and reduce offending. I volunteered to work as an officer-facilitator, in addition to my work as a residential wing officer, on a psychotherapy group. This involves working with a group of eight men; membership changes slowly as each progresses and moves on.

You might think having just expounded these lofty ideals that I am blessed by an aura of vision and assurance in aiming to put theory into practice. Unfortunately not; my own post has proved to be both fascinating and a very hard slog. First, the majority of the inmates on the group, having been guided by a 'civilian' and 'proper therapist', voted with their feet shortly after I'd walked in wearing my prison officer uniform. Nothing in the introduction to therapy books I had read had mentioned this scenario. I sat with the remaining minority. On subsequent groups, exits continued. I almost felt grateful to those remaining if they said anything, let alone anything of therapeutic value. It was a relief after staff group feedbacks to return to the more onerous but simpler task of counting how many prisoners were going out for exercise.

The majority of prisoners at Grendon, and most probably other prisons too, would be deemed too unstable to engage in any psychotherapy groups on the outside. Problems such as too much acting out of hostility and other negative emotions (not to mention a prison number and a catalogue of crimes) would preclude any notion of acceptance on a group. To complicate matters still further, a prison is certainly not the obvious choice for the intimate world of therapy. Prison rules, regimes and restrictions often conflict with the ideals of a therapeutic community, creating its own unique subculture. Some may recall a recently televised series entitled 'The Experiment'. The aim was to recreate a prison, and witness the effects of incarceration upon members of Joe Public. Volunteers, bank managers, brick layers and the like lived this experiment within a specially created 'prison block'. One group became the prisoners, the other the guards (or officers). It soon became apparent that the 'officers', having to assume the role of authority, control and accountability, became more and more insecure in their role, displaying heightened neuroses and eventually ceding their control. Within the other group, the 'prisoners', conversely, many became more confident, deviant and controlling, and effectively defeated the guards. Others became closed down and confused. In the main, though, it seemed that adopting the persona of defiance and deviance was indeed easier and surprisingly authentic under the oppressive conditions of prison. This was played out by a group of men that had tested as being well adjusted, with no history of mental disorder. Imagine then how prison is supposed to affect the ideals of peace, self-acceptance and mental well-being, which is the eventual aim of group psychotherapy – in short, to raise the prisoner's self-esteem, to allow the individual to lead, as the Prison Service doctrine states, law-abiding and useful lives in custody and upon release. If you remember that many of the men suffer severe personality disorders, and indeed us staff have our own quirks and neuroses, it all becomes a minefield.

We staff, a collection of the experienced and inexperienced, with frequent staffing shortages, ask these men to attend a difficult alien experience, namely to attend groups, lower walls built up by years of abuse and self-abuse and to speak their truth – or partial truth – and understanding about their most humiliating and degrading experiences. In short, not only to lose the masks that we all wear, but also to lose the deeply ingrained mask of the long-term criminal, so that collectively each can help the other to address problems and obtain relief.

Trying to understand and work with the behaviour and emotions of these damaged, distressed and dangerous men is often a confusing, overwhelming, but uniquely satisfying process. For the men in prison we are asking them to learn to trust prison officers – authority figures, bearing in mind that their experiences with authority figures from the past (parents, abusers, children's home workers), not forgetting physical fights with prison officers (almost all have had numerous prison sentences), have often been disastrous.

For the men themselves, trying to trust prison staff is thus an unnatural experience. The knock-on effect when the individual finds the courage to speak about painful childhood experiences, a chaotic and unfulfilling life and then revisit the mental disturbance and taboo emotions that exploded at the time of the crime is one of regression. This regression often takes the form of whatever regressive, childlike behaviour the man used as a coping strategy at times of acute stress. It is then that many decide to leave. Why should they put themselves through this, if it makes them feel so lousy? Worse still can be the overload of hearing about everybody else's miserable lives. It is at this stage that some of the obvious differences between those undergoing therapy and stress in a prison, and those undergoing therapy and/or stress on the outside, kick in with a vengeance. At times of stress we seek appropriate or inappropriate sources of comfort and freedom. An individual on the outside can indulge in a little retail therapy, go for a country walk, go to the pub, drive round to see the family, play with the kids, or perhaps go down the converse route and drink too much, take drugs. The positive options of escape and relaxation are largely denied to prisoners. Thus escape, especially when new to the process, involves a regression to past ways of coping with being trapped, depression, drug abuse and isolation. Those with families often succumb to the natural urge to move to a prison closer to home.

Throughout this regression it is expected that each man adheres to the rules of a therapeutic community, namely, taking responsibility for his own actions, challenging, tolerating and understanding the behaviours of others, and taking on practical disciplined roles, attendance, good timekeeping, cleaning, education, even perhaps being the fish tank or finance rep for the wing.

It has increasingly occurred to me that as officers there is no cut-off point from any area of these men's lives, whilst we are trying to make sure they gain all necessary support and attention to help them with the huge responsibilities they face. It soon becomes clear that at Grendon you are entering a parenting, or should I say re-parenting, role, because for the majority of the men their own parents were at best neglectful. We are trying to redress earlier, often disastrous, experiences.

We are parents in the sense that all areas of the prisoners' lives are in one way or another under the control, guidance and oversight of staff. This can be extremely claustrophobic. For example, the first part of the day is spent dealing with complaints about the regime, late unlocks, applications for the doctor, wages checks, and all the unsatisfying minutiae of the complicated running of a complicated red-tape-bound institution. So early mornings can be a struggle, in a not dissimilar way to the rush of mundane issues to be tackled each day in a functioning family household. Certainly a percentage of prisoners will be faking illness, oversleeping, having tantrums. Thus they use similar tactics to schoolchildren or indeed anyone stressed in their workplace, to avoid the perils of the therapy. Accountability for attendance at groups is a mainstay, and it is expected that absences and the underlying reasons for this will be drawn out in therapy (unless many on the group have a large degree of reluctance themselves, which is sometimes the case).

Groups each morning run for an hour and a half. As an officer/facilitator I sit, usually alone, with the eight men on the group. On a good day, if staffing and rotas allow, another officer can join me. The agenda is open-ended. Each man is an individual. All of us have an inbuilt resistance to disclosure in some form or another, and of course rivalries and intolerance present in all groups are often accentuated for these men in this stressful environment, It is commonplace for each to regress to diverting the group, deflecting issues, or just plainly to falsify issues to be seen in a good light (not uncommon human traits!).

Irritability at the inefficiency of prison and its hidebound routines surfaces regularly, especially as a commonly colluded defence to looking at one's own problems. It takes a supreme effort for each to open up to other men that he might even not like. The facilitator or officer on the group subconsciously comes to represent many conscious or subconscious feelings and emotions attached to key people in the men's lives. Thus my own words and non-verbal communications will take on a significance that is unerring. It often feels as if my own mistakes are amplified, at a time when my desire is to help, or challenge and observe in such a way as to get the others to help each other. Similarly, as the facilitator it is all too easy to become the target for hostility when you make an interpretation or observation. This can occur if you have misunderstood, and got it wrong. It can also happen when you have understood a little too well for the other's comfort, and maybe hit the nail on the head, which often draws a hostile response, especially if it confronts an area that the man is desperate to hide. All these issues have meaning, and all are there to be understood.

The experts are the men on the group, who when significantly engaged have a remarkable ability to understand the taboo or upsetting experiences of the man who is using the group on an issue. Of course, sometimes the common bond is too unnerving. We often can't tolerate things in ourselves, so when we see the same taboos in others the temptation is to attack, undermine or repel to get away from that all too real reminder of ourselves.

It is often when tension and negativity exists that we can work as a group to progress, in a not dissimilar way to when in general relationships things come to a head and true feelings are expressed that can bring resolution. My role is to endeavour to bring a space into the group for men to think, and relate to others, rather than just react. The temptation is often to say too much, and try too hard, to resolve things for the men, which prevents themselves drawing upon their own capabilities. A constant worry is that someone will become damaged through the process, and that I might unwittingly add to this damage.

Why do we, staff and inmates, go through this process, if it's all so difficult, you may ask . . . the wages! No, really, the thing that makes it worth it is to see the majority, those who put in the effort, become more outgoing, empathetic and happier. In short, these men get to build on a new potential that has been denied them through years of abuse and the re-enactment of that abuse on the victims of the crimes. For each of us on the group it is harrowing to listen to details of traumatic childhoods and more especially the details of a crime. It is particularly difficult for the men because it takes them back in many cases to their own experiences. However, the underpinning theme of therapy is the understanding of a common bond with others, so that the person who summons up the courage to speak feels this bond, instead of the all too common feeling of alienation.

The whole area is fraught with many blocks, men have to feel safe and trust each other and the facilitator to undergo such work. As with sibling rivalry, some men will push too hard to get their needs met at the cost of the quieter, more withdrawn group member. It usually feels like a difficult juggling game. Certainly, each man will consciously and subconsciously set the scene, and present the challenge for us to listen to and interpret their own world, with the expectation that we can understand, offer relief, and remove and challenge the falsehoods or deceits that they themselves are afraid to confront.

The eventual aim is for all the baggage from the past, once shared and confronted, to be greatly lessened, thus allowing the man to move on from these experiences and look with strength to the future. Men relatively new into therapy find it difficult to accept that disclosure and challenging and understanding others can eventually make them feel better. It is difficult for men used to a lifetime of hiding from and suppressing feelings with drugs or violence to trust this concept. However, men with more experience who are starting to feel better in themselves spend a great deal of time and effort helping to support others to stay.

With regard to the feelings regarding the crime and the victims of crime, the issue is more complex. The heightened empathy that group work often creates means that feelings of remorse, guilt and fellow feeling for what the victim went through are increased. This of course helps reduce risk of further crime and, as the man has learned to understand his emotions and communicate them in a positive way, to build his self-esteem.

So how does it feel to attempt all this as a prison officer? After groups and a wing feedback on each group, many of the men retreat upstairs for their own time. However, this often involves being aware of a fellow group member who has left the group angry, upset and not coping. Much time is given to supporting each other on the landings in this way. It is in these instances that those who cannot communicate their distress are perhaps more at risk.

The same applies to staff. After groups, and collective wing feedbacks from the groups, issued by the inmates, the staff group meet to feed back the substance of the groups, to gain advice and, if time allows, share some of the pressures of trying to coordinate and listen to difficult material. If some of this difficult material echoes your own experiences in life then trying to facilitate a group is particularly draining. Under these circumstances staff have to maintain a professional and silent front, with the pressure of not leaking or divulging any of your own discomfort or life experiences. This gets easier with practice, and usually it is very easy to make mistakes here and get drawn in. However, the men need to be free of the staff member's own frailties, to assume that the facilitator is both impartial and strong enough not to be directly affected by whatever they divulge. This additional pressure usually catches up with staff if they are not aware of it. Consequences can include strong negative transferences of unspoken feelings, and stress levels that can rise off the Richter scale.

It is then that it is necessary to share these problems. Unfortunately the time constraints mean that each staff member can easily neglect to ask for help and supervision from colleagues. Feelings can easily be suppressed as calls over prison radios call for staff to man the exercise yard, and assemble to count inmates off to exercise. The change in role from facilitator to officer is quite stark. The moving from the personal to the all encompassing structure of a multitude of protracted practical problems, e.g. shortages in prisoners' moneys, paperwork being delayed or lost, regime changes and so on, allows no time for reflection. The feeling is akin to walking out of a disturbing and powerful film at the cinema into the bright lights and bustle of a busy city street. A front has to be put up, and there is often an escape into overactivity or humour as a defence against your feelings. The change for inmates too must be somewhat unnerving: one minute a man is divulging issues he hasn't wanted to admit even to himself; shortly afterwards you are giving the man a rub-down search as he leaves the wing for exercise! This is not an experience replicated in any therapy group outside of prison.

The distinctions between therapy and prison life in a prison therapeutic community are impervious. The pressure of group work takes its toll on men who often have limited social skills and intolerance without this added pressure of trying to make sense of therapy and undertake to change. Many of the pressures experienced in groups are translated into antisocial forms of behaviour off groups until the men learn more positive coping strategies of asking for help. Staff help isn't always available, due to other demands on their time. Similarly, it is often felt more helpful if the men learn to contain their anxieties, or ask other inmates for help. Otherwise there is a risk of overload for staff or of simply getting too drawn into a particular man's world, thus becoming the focus for attention and advice rather than the group, which is indeed problematic. It is a trap that is not always easy to avoid.

Behaviour off groups is observed and noted by staff and inmates alike. It goes without saying that much behaviour on the prison landings where the cells are located, an area often away from the scrutiny of staff, goes underground. It is a frequent complaint by the men that their peer group members often speak and behave differently when feeling not under pressure to please staff. However, it is difficult for all behaviour of both staff and inmates to be consistently hidden from others. It is expected that there are no secrets in a therapeutic community. However, those men who have their cover blown by another bringing these issues to the group or wing, after a show of hostility or denial, normally learn and gain support from the experience, usually after much lively debate, and a degree of 'staff bashing'. Staff bashing is a common occurrence, whereby men publicise the shortcomings of staff, either collectively or individually, to avoid looking at and taking responsibility for their own behaviour. Conversely, as the men gain confidence in their own abilities they become increasingly aware that their understanding, not only of group dynamics but also of the issues and decisions regarding the management of the wing, is often superior to the capabilities of staff. It is at this point that those who are engaged in the process can make a real difference to the community and, in so doing, gain personal benefit. Of course, with increased vision comes the understandable resentment of having to be at times dependent on staff decisions and inconsistencies. However, there is also the awareness in the more reflective men that staff have a greater access to private and security information and need at times to be the final decision makers. The ability to work through and tolerate these contradictions is good practice for the balancing of freedom and constraints in the outside world.

It can be tempting for inmates to forget that the skills gained in therapy in this unnatural environment are necessary for release. I have lost count of the number of times that I have heard prisoners argue that the issues that come up on groups and in the wing have no relevance to the outside world. It is at this point the next statement is usually, 'My behaviour will be completely different on the outside.'

Of course, to an extent it will be, because nothing will quite replicate the unique culture of a prison. However, behaviour in groups is to a certain extent universal, as we are social animals and can learn and be challenged on our habitual ways of behaving and reacting. The aim is for each to become more confident and open, taking risks to communicate to others, gain and give support, to learn trust and to progress. After innumerable ups and downs this happens for those who 'put the work in'. It is specifically for the outside world that these hopefully gained skills will be tested. Within prison, in spite of all the recurrent frustrations of being inside, there are advantages. Company, inclusion, a shared experience, no bills and the necessities of life (though obviously very basic) are provided. The practice of deliberating over decisions for other prisoners, voting for or against them being given a new job or the chance of a day out on temporary release, or whether an inmate should incur a penalty to an extent replicates the decision-making and balancing act we make for family members and friends and associates on the outside. In short, the practice of how to gain responsibility, or gain help.

In contrast, the very real worry about securing employment and accommodation on the outside weighs heavily on most. Almost all are institutionalised, and are trying by the above methods to break away from this. However, it is still a frightening prospect for most to leave. In other prisons or upon release the majority are aware that they will miss the close emotional contact and support of the other men and staff on the wing. Many will be returning to the home area that presented the hazards and temptations that helped the individual on the path to offending in the first place. Contributory difficulties and issues with family members can still exist. For those moving to new areas or other prisons, the fear of loneliness, isolation and reverting back to form as a result are also prevalent. Will the strength gained in therapy be enough not only to help with these potential pressures, but also to allow the man peace of mind and the ability to progress and enjoy life? This, of course, is the million-dollar question.

Staff and the inmates get used to watching, observing and at times worrying about each man's behaviour. The bulk of the time at staff meetings is really apportioned in one way or another to this. A feeling of pride exists in staff, especially those with a personal responsibility for a particular inmate, if the man is progressing, even in small ways. Conversely, frustrations and worries mount if someone is going downhill. The challenge here is to understand and work with this common process. It is obvious to each of us how we become personally involved in each man's ups and downs, and at times are protective of the particular men that we bear personal responsibility for, counteracting criticism from other staff, and agonising over disappointments and decisions. Although each of us would be hard pushed to admit it, such tendencies can be counter-productive, and it is then when we need the impartiality of other staff. The inmates often joke that our meetings are just a forum for coffee and biscuits – and of course those two ingredients are vital.

The point of all these deliberations is to build up an idea of how each man is going to cope on the outside. Will he do OK? Vitally, will there be no more victims? We all have an awareness how easily risk factors inherent in society and each individual can present themselves, with the end result being another terrible crime, another victim dead or perhaps ruined for life. Many of these men will again resume the responsibilities of parenthood; with the abounding hope held by all that this time they will make a success of it. If not, will these children end up in prison?

Both staff and inmates are not totally isolated from these real issues in prison. Not only do concerns and issues about family members permeate each group, we get to meet and see these homes and people with the men themselves. All prisons have visiting facilities. Grendon offers family days whereby family members spend a day on the wing, hosted mainly by the prisoners, and are free to use the time to get to know each other and recognise changes – and unfortunately problems too. These issues are, it is hoped, talked about in the groups.

The most dramatic departures from the norm for both staff and inmates alike, however, are days out. Each man can after a year in therapy apply for a day out, escorted by one or two wing staff to visit family members at the family home. Others may be rushed to a hospital bed if a close relative is dying. It is a release, literally and psychologically, for men and staff to drive away from the prison to gain a snapshot of the family home for a day. It is also an emotionally charged day! Both the man and staff member will have had to go through a long and tortuous process to get clearance from other staff and inmates, not to mention security and the financiers before it all starts – and then there's the paperwork!

The security rating of many of the men means that they will have to be handcuffed to a prison officer for the duration of the day. Some feel that the prospect of sitting in the family living room under these circumstances is just too much and decline the chance. For us staff whilst the process of sitting in a car, seeing motorways and new areas is hardly life-changing, suddenly being in a family's front room, cuffed to their husband, son, father or brother is a strange experience. We are at once privy to their private world, but a somewhat unnatural addition. There's also awareness that for the man himself and family members, this is a culture shock. It is strange for us to be removed from the claustrophobic world of the prison to looking at photos and ornaments and being offered sandwiches, cake and all the trappings of domesticity. We are used to hearing about the relevance of these people and their issues and surroundings on the therapy groups in a prison wing. On the wing you can only imagine the surroundings, the personalities and their relevance to these men, their lives, and of course all these seemingly ordinary details, sometimes depressingly ordinary, formed part of the tapestry to the backdrop to the crime. With handcuffs and uniforms we, too, are a visible reminder of the crime. It again reinforces for me that there is no cut-off point for us from these men's lives. This is a powerful and absorbing feeling.

Both we and the man himself are evaluating the day. For us – is the family pleased to see the man? Does it seem like a hazardous environment, one where the prisoner and his family look as if it is possible to make a successful go of things? Are they able to communicate over problems, even allowing for our presence? The prisoner himself is usually increasingly nervous on the journey. The fantasy for many months or years is that all will be happy, that tensions will vanish and that the fantasy will not turn out to be dashed by a negative outcome. The visit is only a starting point, but signals to an extent the state of things to come, so it is an important day. Does it mark the start of a new beginning, or are there uncomfortable echoes of the past for one or both sides? All this will hopefully get debated on the groups, although men are naturally defensive over negative personal issues, and it takes courage to overcome this.

Those on a determinate sentence will progress after this initial visit to spending four or five days away from the prison at a time, at the family home, if they have one or if they are intending to return to it. Others will acclimatise themselves to pre-release hostels, before their permanent release.

It is a strange feeling seeing a man leave the prison for the outside world or, in the case of lifers, the move to another prison. Before this time you have had a part in most areas of their lives, as have the other staff and men on the wing. We leave for home each evening, but the prisoners stay. Mistakes can be rectified. We get to know each other very well. There is a common bond of purpose, and a great deal of humour and good feeling that I have neglected to mention throughout this chapter. Perhaps because we take it for granted. The next minute he is leaving. On release he could be sat in the pub in a few hours' time, but hopefully not getting blasted. He will be walking in the park, or sat alone with his worries. He will be a citizen. Each and every prisoner that we meet in prison states that this sentence is his last sentence. It is our collective responsibility to try and ensure this is the case. As often as not we have our fingers crossed!

Chapter 12

The concept of dangerousness and younger people

Celia Taylor

Introduction

The peak frequency for inflicting physical aggression upon others occurs surprisingly young – at two years old.[1] This does not alarm us, because a key factor that we weigh up when assessing dangerousness is the capability of an individual of inflicting real harm. The risks are much higher when a child reaches adolescence, the peak age for offending in general.[2] But, despite the widespread fear of crime, teenage delinquency is largely directed at property, and while the damage done has a high nuisance value and is not so 'petty' to its victims, it is seen as part of adolescence and assumed – correctly – that most kids will 'grow out of it'. Occasionally, however, a crime is committed by a young person that leads to near universal horror, fear and rejection. The same British examples of this phenomenon in recent decades are always cited, since they remain so alive in the public memory: Mary Bell, who was convicted at the age of 11 of the manslaughter of two small boys; and the ten-year-old killers of James Bulger, who were captured on video leading the toddler out of a shopping mall and away from his mother to a nearby railway track, where his mutilated dead body was later found. Such behaviour by children remains rare, and is widely judged to be due to the perpetrators' 'inherent evil' – and thus both unforgivable and immutable – rather than the circumstances of their formative years.

Young people achieve adult maturity and responsibility over time as part of a gradual developmental process. This is reflected in a variety of legal milestones: in England a child can stop attending school, and consent to sexual intercourse and marriage at 16. At 17 he or she can drive a car, and at 18 vote, although many young people still celebrate their 21st birthday as their true 'coming of age'. Abstract thinking is developed and refined, such that the hypothetical and the general can be considered, rather than merely the concrete and particular; hence the teenager's penchant for idealism and debates about political and moral mores. Piaget[3] termed this the move from *concrete operations* to *formal operations*, but his assumption that this was normally achieved by the age of 14 has been disproved by a number of studies[4] showing that a significant proportion of adults are still functioning at the level of concrete operations. Since individual youngsters vary so widely as to how cognitively and emotionally ready they are to meet their life circumstances – which, for some, are appallingly difficult – it has been argued that, at 10, the age of criminal responsibility is both too low and too inflexible.

Adolescents face a rapid growth in height whilst developing an adult sexual physique; coping with these obvious changes can bring anxieties about performance and looks such as sometimes lead to profound self-doubt. Meanwhile, adolescents also have to negotiate first dates, acceptance by their peer group and the discovery of a solid sense of self. This is a traditional time for experimentation, and choices have been increased by the sexual, women's and gay liberation movements on the one hand, and the growth in children's rights (with legal limits set upon, for example, adult violence towards them) on the other. Despite the popular conception of a 'loss of deference', and the stereotype of adolescents challenging authority, it has long been established that most teenagers get on well with their parents[5] and agree with them on fundamental moral or political issues.[6] Thus it seems that most adolescents evolve into reasonably well-adjusted adults. What, then, is different about dangerous young people?

A developmental understanding of dangerous behaviour

With recent reports showing that violent crime has doubled in England and Wales,[7] there is currently a huge political emphasis on detecting and preventing the risk of serious offending. The focus is particularly upon personality disorder, because these individuals are more likely to commit violent crimes, and fill our prisons.[8] Adult antisocial personality disorder (APD) has long been known to have its roots in childhood delinquency,[9] and violent behaviour from a young age is one of the most significant warning signs for violence in an older child or teenager. From recent research into known risk factors (*see* Box 12.1), it is possible to propose a developmental pathway as to how and why young people become dangerous.

Box 12.1   Risk factors for antisocial personality disorder

Neurobiological factors
- Genetic[10] and gene–environment interactions[11]
- Neuroanatomical and neurophysiological abnormalities[12]
- Autonomic hypoarousal when anticipating adverse stimuli[13]
- Neutral processing of emotionally charged words and events[14,15]

Individual factors
- Personality[16]
- Early onset of frequent and varied antisocial behaviour[17]

- Childhood abuse or neglect[18]
- Conduct disorder co-morbid with anxiety, depression and substance misuse[17]

Family factors
- Parenting style of harsh and inconsistent discipline; poor parental supervision[19]
- Parental criminality[20] and psychopathology[21]
- Avoidant or disorganised attachment style[22]
- Witnessing violence between parents[23]
- Parental separation/divorce[20]

Socio-economic factors
- Low family socio-economic status[20]
- Large income gap between rich and poor[24]

Peer group
- Peer delinquency[25]

The most vulnerable children are likely to face multiple risk factors at all levels, none of which individually 'causes' APD, but which interact in a cumulative way over time. Thus, poverty alone is not a risk factor until combined with, say, abuse, family breakdown, an impulsive temperament and adverse peer group pressures. It is not known which of the risk factors listed are necessary and/or sufficient. The picture that emerges from these studies of the development of personality disorder is one of a *hierarchical developmental model*,[17] in which a relatively high proportion of boys show early onset of aggressive behaviour, but only a proportion go on to develop conduct disorder; out of these, only about a third will go on to develop APD as adults. It is likely that those most frequently and severely affected by the above risk factors will show the most dangerous behaviour at the youngest ages.[26] APD, according to DSM-IV criteria, is not diagnosable before the age of 18, when personality is deemed to be fully formed; in recognition of the very real threat posed by sometimes much younger individuals, however, a Youth Version of the Hare Psychopathy Checklist (PCL-YV) – which assesses a similar concept and incorporates a measure of severity – has been validated for adolescent offenders.[27]

Studies of the risk factors for borderline personality disorder (BPD)[28] also show a history of neurological difficulties, poor impulse control and conduct disorder to be common, while first degree relatives are more likely to have BPD themselves. Other studies have found a high prevalence of early losses and separations.[29] There has been a growing realisation in recent years of the role of chronic childhood trauma, particularly sexual abuse, in the origins of BPD.[30] Approximately 60% of patients report such a history, but it appears that it is its *combination* with parental neglect and chaotic or inconsistent home environments that lead to borderline symptoms in adulthood.

A developmental understanding of dangerous minds

Our perceptions of dangerousness, both public and professional, tend to neglect the concept of the dangerous mind. Most risk assessment tools emphasise overtly violent or irresponsible behaviour, but ignore (with the exception of the PCL) the qualities of emotion and thought so memorably described by Cleckley[31] such as shamelessness, an incapacity for love, and an overriding tendency to project blame onto others. These mental characteristics, it could be argued, are even more ominous than manifest delinquency in young people, since they underpin the plotting, sadism and ruthlessness that precede acts of the most serious harm. These are also the qualities that we tend to assume others *do not* have, leading to a potentially serious underestimation of risk. In a society that idealises children, they are especially not attributed to the young, which may explain the subsequent demonisation of individuals like Mary Bell, mentioned above. Very few large studies have attempted to measure the emergence of these more hidden 'symptoms' of APD during childhood. An exception was the Pittsburgh Youth Study, which found that parents' and teachers' report of boys' lack of guilt was one of the strongest factors associated with serious delinquency.[32]

Any professional seeking to treat young people who have been or might be dangerous will inevitably be drawn away from a consideration of broad risk factors, to listening to an account of each individual's experiences. Youngsters want, as best they can, to tell their story and, above all, to find *meaning* in it. This is important therapeutically, because dangerous acts are preceded by dangerous thoughts, feelings and interpretations of the intentions of others that directly resonate with how that young person has been treated in the past. Clinicians working in forensic settings will be aware that it is the pain of damaging past relationships that remains so alive, and that tends to get acted out in the present day.

Much is now known about the biological and emotional effects of trauma upon the growing mind.[33] One of the most important functions of the mother or care-giver is that of enabling the young child to develop a reflective function or capacity to 'mentalize'.[34] Maltreatment undermines this capacity for acquiring a theory of mind, either because the child cannot bear to know of the hatred and cruelty in the mind of its parent, or because of the inherent confusion produced when the parent's stated intentions (often presented as loving and in the interests of the child) contradict their abusive actions. The results include difficulties with emotional self-awareness, with perceiving and understanding of the emotions of others, and with the ability to regulate levels of arousal.

Physical, sexual or emotional abuse occurring at an older age, and often lasting for years, leads to further distortions of the developing personality. The abused young person is likely to develop a strong sense of being worthless: damaged goods to be used or abused at will by others. He or she will expect boundaries to be violated and his or her own perception of, and reaction to, reality to be invalidated or ignored. The painful memories and other intrusive post-traumatic symptoms that result from such experiences cannot be processed or integrated into a coherent, or acceptable, sense of identity; instead, they are relived, sometimes literally, with the young person either in the role of repeated victim, or identifying with the aggressor.[35] Adolescence is a particularly vulnerable period: as noted above, teenagers are highly sensitive and self-conscious about their maturing bodies in particular, and an experience of being belittled, mocked or humiliated can lead to profound and destructive rage.[36] Unable to express this rage symbolically through language or fantasy, young men are particularly prone to concrete acts of violence, the unconscious intent behind which is to 'kill off' the one who 'sees' their shame. Young women, on the other hand, more often express self-loathing and anger through acts of self-harm, although these gender distinctions are by no means absolute.

Treatment

There are currently few treatment opportunities for dangerous young people unless they have a serious psychotic illness, and many therefore spend years in custody. Within the health service, one ward at Broadmoor maximum secure hospital provides a range of therapies to young people, but, given the nature of the institution and increasing pressure on beds, only those who have already committed a crime of the utmost gravity are accepted.

Given this lack of provision, there is a new major policy drive on the part of the government to develop a full range of services.[37] My experience has been on a personality disorder unit (PDU) at the medium secure level. Here, admission to hospital can interrupt offending that is escalating in its seriousness, *before* a young person has done something irrevocably damaging or even fatal. Typical crimes committed by patients admitted to the PDU include arson, assault, stalking, threats to kill and hostage-taking. Increasingly, young people are referred whose deliberate self-harm is severe, repetitive and out of control. These individuals pose a dilemma, since ostensibly they do not pose a danger to others and it could be argued that medium secure conditions are over-restrictive and unnecessary. However, this level of self-harm is often associated with repeated absconding and suicide attempts that general psychiatric wards cannot contain, as well as, in my experience, secret but strong urges to attack others.

All patients are detained under the Mental Health Act via civil or court-imposed orders, but this does not mean that therapy is 'forced' upon them: allowing for ambivalence and unconscious, repeated attempts to be rejected, each actually wants to be on the Unit. It could even be argued that patients' legal detention provides them with a degree of long-term security and stability they have hitherto lacked. It is true that each is carefully selected for a willingness to engage in treatment, a degree of psychological curiosity about themselves, and a wish to change the patterns of destructive and hurtful behaviour that have hitherto characterised their lives. Above all, patients who come to the Unit want to be taken seriously: 'I'm afraid I'm going to kill someone one day' is a commonly expressed anxiety. Such statements, as well as the behaviour that has led to the referral, should be recognised as an expression of hope that someone will listen.[38]

> **Clinical vignette**
>
> Annabel, aged 19 and the only daughter of middle class parents, had first started self-harming three years earlier. This behaviour had become compulsive, and included scalding, cutting, head-banging and tying ligatures around her neck. Despite considerable efforts, her local general psychiatric hospital had been unable to prevent her from running away on several occasions. This was extremely anxiety-provoking for the staff, since she had made numerous suicidal threats and attempts. Usually, however, she would abscond back to her parents' house, particularly after she had self-harmed in a very visible way, such as on her face. On the last such occasion she set a fire whilst the family was out, causing thousands of pounds of damage. Following admission to the Personality Disorder Unit, Annabel's self-harm continued, frequently leading to her being nursed on enhanced levels of observation. She eventually asked to be secluded, expressing a fear that she would attack the (female) deputy charge nurse for reasons she found hard to explain.

Perhaps the first task following a patient's admission is to foster safe attachments: these are relatively rare in the childhood experiences of forensic patients,[39] but are essential in promoting the individual's ability to cope with anxiety and distress.[40] One function of Annabel's self-harm was that it ensured the close proximity and supervision of the nursing staff, which in itself helped to reduce her anxiety. Over time, the nursing staff can teach strategies for managing thoughts of self-harm, such as listening to music or playing Scrabble; for young people a PlayStation is a particularly successful distraction. During a community meeting Annabel's peers made it clear that they suffered from, and disliked, seeing the results of her self-harm – especially since, after she scalded herself with a mixture of boiling water and sugar, the dining room was locked off and their free access to drinks curtailed.

Self-harm can also be a form of communication, since patients also find it very difficult to name their emotions, or to speak of them with someone else. This is especially true of negative feelings that threaten to overwhelm, especially when these are directed towards someone who 'should be' – and is, in part – a loved one. The significance of Annabel's impulse to assault the deputy charge nurse was that this member of staff, with whom she had initially formed a close, needy relationship, was leaving. This kind of 'toxic' attachment early on in the admission can provide not only a clue to the individual's attachment style, but a warning of possible violence.[41] Annabel's true rage and fear of abandonment lay with her mother, who had frequently left her in the charge of a stepfather who sexually abused her, although knowing about such feelings at a conscious level induced profound guilt: like most children, she had protected her mother by assuming her own badness and deservingness of her fate.[42]

As mentioned above, secure attachments are also the starting point for the capacity to imagine other people's feelings and states of mind,[34] thus promoting empathy and reducing the risk of violence. Closely related is the ability to express one's own state of mind symbolically, rather than in concrete action, which many offenders lack. Not unusually, Annabel, who also suffered from dyslexia, found this less threatening to do during art therapy: since shame and aggression are projected into images rather than solely the therapist, their intensity is ameliorated.

Clinical vignette

At the age of 16, Rick took his foster-parents hostage and threatened to kill them. His biological father had abandoned his mother when Rick was a baby, and although she quickly found a new partner, he was a violent alcoholic recently thrown out of the army. As a result, Rick grew up experiencing extreme intimidation. Whilst in custody on remand he assaulted a prison officer, following which he attempted to hang himself with his bedsheets.

Once admitted to the Unit, Rick had difficulty forming attachments with staff: he had a fear, of which he was profoundly ashamed, of sleeping in his room at night in case they mounted an attack for which he was unprepared. He took to placing his belt under his pillow, to use as a weapon should he need one. Rick had a strong and tenacious identification with a terrorising abuser, who cruelly prolonged his victims' wait for an assault they knew was bound to come. This scenario was repeated time and again on the ward, with Rick provoking the nursing staff into stand-offs which necessarily ended in him being restrained. Paradoxically, this was the outcome he was unconsciously seeking: to be physically controlled, but only when his anticipation was at fever pitch. He referred to himself as an 'adrenaline junkie', while the staff felt abused themselves and began to resent being turned from helpers into enforcers. These feelings were compounded when Rick made complaints about them to the Advocacy Service, members of which tended to see him purely as the victim of a brutalising regime.

The situation was resolved – fortuitously rather than by design – when Rick was allocated a primary nurse who was himself ex-army. This individual's background of itself won Rick's grudging respect, but it was his skilful use of his personality as a tool,[43] judging when to empathise and when to confront, that awoke Rick's sense of responsibility towards others.

The institution and young people

Young people detained in secure facilities for treatment have many of the risk factors for suicide:[44] they are mostly single, unemployed and have almost universally experienced childhood deprivation, abuse and disrupted relationships. They require long-term treatment and frequently exhibit challenging behaviour. Finally, they often have additional problems with depression, substance misuse and deliberate self-harm. These young people are highly sensitive to comparisons, which they themselves make, with others of their age: often nursed by staff not much older than they, who can visibly hold down a job, own a car and go on holidays, it is not difficult to see how envy and past experiences of failure can lead to despair. Young people have a need to be respected and believed in, especially when they cannot do this for themselves.

For treatment to be successful, the institution within which young people are detained must demonstrate a commitment to the task, as well as a self-monitoring function to ensure that this commitment is adhered to. Two areas are of particular importance.

1   The provision of skilled staff who are willing and able to stay the course. This involves offering a high standard of training which must be ongoing, as well as staff supervision and support. A particularly stressful aspect of the work is the profound tendency of patients to perceive all help as abuse;[43] thus small errors and failings are taken to be signs of cruelty and neglect, and staff are roundly accused of such. Not unnaturally, these genuinely dedicated individuals increasingly resent their good intentions being misperceived as the opposite; this is one of the main reasons that personality-disordered individuals tend, over time, to become seen as evil, or 'just thugs' as one nurse said to me, while their inner pain and loneliness are overlooked. Staff of all disciplines need both opportunity and permission honestly to express emotions, such as anger and frustration, that run counter to their professional self-image, since this capacity to make others feel bad about themselves is one of their patients' core problems.

2   The institution must also provide young people with opportunities for normal life, both inside and outside its locked doors. Examples in my hospital include the chance to beat another ward's team in football, and trips out to the local cinema (where the risk assessment permits) so that they are not entirely isolated from the popular culture the rest of their age group enjoys. Patients who cook during occupational therapy sessions are encouraged to share the meal with their peers, and the kitchens provide a cake for the ward party on birthdays. Forensic institutions are particularly prone to deal with anxiety by the enforcement of petty rules and a regimented regime.[45] Although these youngsters do need structure and containment, this should never stand in the way of flexibility and creativity.

Finally, young people need goals: 'what do I have to do to get out of here?' is a common and legitimate question, which forces the institution and its professionals to be specific about the kind of progress they are looking for, how it can be achieved, and over what anticipated timescale. It is surprising how many will understand an answer, not just at the concrete behavioural level, but at the psychological level too.

References

1   Tremblay R, Boulerice B, Harden P et al. (1996) Do children in Canada become more aggressive as they approach adolescence? In: Human Resources Development Canada & Statistics Canada (eds) *Growing Up*

in Canada: National Longitudinal Survey of Children and Youth. Statistics Canada, Ottawa.

2 Farrington D (1986) Stepping stones to adult criminal careers. In: D Olweus, J Block and M Radke-Yarrow (eds) *Development of Antisocial and Prosocial Behaviour.* Academic Press, New York.

3 Piaget J (1966) *The Growth of Logical Thinking.* Routledge and Kegan Paul, London.

4 Neimark E (1975) Intellectual development during adolescence. In: F Horowitz (ed.) *Review of Child Development Research*, Vol. 4. University of Chicago Press, Chicago.

5 Ghodsian M and Lambert L (1978) Mum and Dad are not so bad: views of sixteen-year-olds on how they get on with their parents. *J Assoc Educ Psychol.* **4**: 27–33.

6 Gustafson B (1972) *Life Values of High School Youth in Sweden.* Institute of Sociology of Religion, Stockholm.

7 Office for National Statistics (1996) *Notifiable Offences Recorded by Police: England and Wales* (abstract of statistics). Office for National Statistics, London.

8 Coid J (2003) Formulating strategies for the prevention of violent behaviour: 'high risk' or 'population' strategies? In: D Farrington and J Coid (eds) *Early Prevention of Antisocial Behaviour.* Cambridge University Press, Cambridge.

9 Robins L (1966) *Deviant Children Grown Up: a sociological and psychiatric study of sociopathic personality.* Williams and Wilkins, Baltimore.

10 McGuffin P, Moffitt T and Thapar A (2002) Personality disorders. In: P McGuffin, M Owen and I Gottesman (eds) *Psychiatric Genetics and Genomics.* Oxford University Press, Oxford.

11 Reiss D, Hetherington E, Plomin R *et al.* (1995) Genetic questions for environmental studies: differential parenting and psychopathology in adolescence. *Archives of General Psychiatry.* **52**: 925–36.

12 Siever L (1998) Neurobiology in psychopathy. In: T Millon, E Simonsen, M Birket-Smith *et al.* (eds) *Psychopathy: antisocial, criminal and violent behaviour.* The Guilford Press, New York.

13 Brennan P, Raine A, Schulsinger F *et al.* (1997) Psychophysiological protective factors for male subjects at high risk for criminal behaviour. *American Journal of Psychiatry.* **154**: 853–5.

14 Williamson S, Harpur T and Hare R (1991) Abnormal processing of affective words by psychopaths. *Psychophysiology.* **28**(3): 260–73.

15 Patrick C, Bradley M and Lang P (1993) Emotion in the criminal psychopath: startle reflex modulation. *Journal of Abnormal Psychology.* **102**(1): 82–92.

16 Shiner R and Caspi A (2003) Personality differences in childhood and adolescence: measurement, development and consequences. *Journal of Child Psychology and Psychiatry.* **44**: 2–32.

17 Loeber R, Green S and Lahey B (2003) Risk factors for adult antisocial personality. In: D Farrington and J Coid (eds) *Early Prevention of Adult Antisocial Behaviour.* Cambridge University Press, Cambridge.

18 Lunts B and Widom C (1994) Antisocial personality disorder in abused and neglected children grown up. *American Journal of Psychiatry.* **151**: 670–4.

19 Farrington D (1995) The development of offending and antisocial behaviour from childhood: key findings from the Cambridge Study in Delinquent Development. *Journal of Child Psychology and Psychiatry.* **36**: 929–64.

20 Farrington D (2000) Families and crime. In: J Wilson and J Petersilia (eds) *Crime: public policies for crime control.* Institute for Contemporary Studies, Oakland, CA.

21 Livesley W (2003) The origins of personality disorder. In: W Livesley (ed.) *Practical Management of Personality Disorder.* The Guilford Press, New York.

22 de Zulueta F (1993) Theories of aggression and violence. In: C Cordess and M Cox (eds) *Forensic Psychotherapy: crime, psychodynamics and the offender patient.* Jessica Kingsley Publishers Ltd, London.

23 Grych J and Fincham F (1990) Marital conflict and children's adjustment: a cognitive-context framework. *Psychological Bulletin.* **108**: 267–90.

24 Kawachi I and Kennedy B (1997) Socio-economic determinants of health: health and social cohesion: why care about income inequality? *BMJ.* **314**: 1037–40.

25 Hawkins J, Herrenkohl T, Farrington D *et al.* (1998) A review of predictors of youth violence. In: R Loeber and D Farrington (eds) *Serious and Violent Juvenile Offenders.* Sage, Thousand Oaks, CA.

26 Vitelli R (1997) Comparison of early and late start models of delinquency in adult offenders. *International Journal of Offender Therapy and Comparative Criminology.* **41**: 351–7.

27 Forth A, Kosson D and Hare R (2003) *The Hare Psychopathy Checklist: Youth Version.* Multi-Health Systems, Toronto.

28 Gabbard G (2000) Cluster B personality disorders: borderline. In: *Psychodynamic Psychiatry in Clinical Practice.* American Psychiatric Press, Washington, DC.

29 Zanarini M and Frankenburg F (1997) Pathways to the development of borderline personality disorder. *Journal of Personality Disorders.* **11**: 93–104.

30 Zanarini M, Williams A, Lewis R *et al.* (1997) Reported pathological childhood experiences associated with the development of borderline personality disorder. *American Journal of Psychiatry.* **154**: 1101–6.

31 Cleckley H (1941) *The Mask of Sanity.* CV Mosby, St Louis, MO.

32 Loeber R, Farrington D, Stouthamer-Loeber M *et al.* (1998) *Antisocial Behaviour and Mental Health Problems: explanatory factors in childhood and adolescence.* Lawrence Erlbaum, Mahweh, NJ.

33 van der Kolk B (1996) The body keeps the score: approaches to the psychobiology of post-traumatic stress disorder. In: B van der Kolk, A McFarlane and L Weisaeth (eds) *Traumatic Stress: the effects of overwhelming experience on mind, body and society.* The Guilford Press, New York.

34 Fonagy P, Gergely G, Jurist E *et al.* (2002) *Affect Regulation, Mentalization, and the Development of the Self.* Other Press, New York.

35 Freud A (1936) *The Ego and the Mechanisms of Defence.* Hogarth Press, London.

36 Gilligan J (1996) Exploring shame in special settings. In: C Cordess and M Cox (eds) *Forensic Psychotherapy: crime, psychodynamics and the offender patient.* Jessica Kingsley Publishers Ltd, London.

37 National Institute for Mental Health in England (2003) *Personality Disorder: no longer a diagnosis of exclusion.* Department of Health, London.

38 Winnicott D (1986) Delinquency as a sign of hope. In: D Winnicott (ed.) *Home Is Where We Start From.* Penguin Books, London.

39 Frodi A, Dernevik M, Sepa A *et al.* (2001) Current attachment representations of incarcerated offenders varying in degree of psychopathy. *Attachment and Human Development.* **3**: 269–83.

40 Bowlby J (1988) *Attachment and Loss. Vol. 3: Loss.* Hogarth Press, London (1988 edn, Pimlico, London).

41 Adshead G (2002) Three degrees of security: attachment and forensic institutions. *Criminal Behaviour and Mental Health.* **12**: S31–S45.

42 Fairburn W (1952) *Psychoanalytic Studies of the Personality.* Routledge and Kegan Paul, London.

43 Hinshelwood R (2002) Abusive help – helping abuse: the psychodynamic impact of severe personality disorder on caring institutions. *Criminal Behaviour and Mental Health.* **12**: S20–S30.

44 Gordon H (2002) Suicide in secure psychiatric facilities. *Advances in Psychiatric Treatment.* **8**: 408–17.

45 Murphy D (2002) Risk assessment as collective clinical judgement. *Criminal Behaviour and Mental Health.* **12**: 169–78.

Chapter 13

Where lies the danger? A psychodrama approach

Jinnie Jeffries

It is a Tuesday afternoon. George is held by each ankle as he watches someone in the role of his father return from the pub and order his son, George (held by a group member), to take off his vest and lean over the couch. George's father then takes off his belt and thrashes the chair that represents the child's back. He listens to his own screams and struggles to get free to remove the belt from his father's hand and rescue himself from the nightly ritual of abuse and violence and the internal father figure that dominates his adult life. His only crime at the age of seven was to be an unwanted child who restricted his father's activity and trapped him in a hapless marriage. His mother out at work could not ignore the welts on the child's back but did little to protect her son from the nightly abuse. George is serving a life sentence for manslaughter.

As a psychodrama psychotherapist at HMP Grendon, I am familiar with working with dangerous people, those who are serving a sentence for rape, murder and assault and those who have inflicted abuse and violence as parents, family friends and custodians on those I have been employed to work with. I regard the second category as being as dangerous as the first in that even though they have not been brought to justice they continue to motivate crimes of violence and assault as part of the internal world of the offender. It is my intention here to convey how these early, often disruptive, abusive and violent relationships play a part in criminal behaviour and how psychodrama attempts to resolve some of the hatred and sense of abuse that frequently gets displaced onto innocent victims.

Psychodynamic theory

The work of John Bowlby, Mary Ainsworth and Mary Maine has contributed to our understanding of how the quality of early attachment relationships and good parenting influence our view of ourselves, of the other and of the world in which we live and how these early experiences and the kinds of attachments created are crucial to development of the personality.

If all goes well in these early developmental years we grow up feeling secure and trusting of others. We are able to make and maintain healthy relationships and deal with difficulties as and when they arrive without too much distress or dysfunction. By things going well it means that the significant others who are responsible for our emotional well-being provide a safe enough environment which in turn provides a secure base and 'working models' or maps, which enable us to deal with the world in which we find ourselves. 'Good parenting enables us to trust and explore our environment based on a sense of coherence and personal integration.'[1] 'The attachment dynamic' is not confined to childhood but continues throughout life.[2]

Research supporting Bowlby's theories indicates that many individuals suffering from anxiety and insecurity or showing signs of dependency, immaturity and low self-image have been exposed to pathogenic parenting. This exposure results in unconscious resentment persisting in later life, usually expressed away from the parents towards someone weaker.[3] In studying the effects on personality development in children who have been assaulted physically and psychologically, Martin Rodeheffer found that they were depressed, passive and inhibited but also angry and aggressive.[4] Bowlby's observations of young children who had been ill-treated and abused showed with unmistakable clarity how early in life certain characteristic patterns of behaviour become established. 'A significant proportion of rejected and abused children grow up to perpetuate the cycle of family violence by continuing to respond in social situations with the very same patterns of behaviour.'[5]

Likewise Bion's notion of 'maternal containment'[6] has gained widespread acceptance within the psychoanalytic world, as has Winnicott's description of the 'good enough mother' whose role is to contain the infant's 'unthinkable anxieties' and transform them into manageable emotions that can later be integrated into the child's developing ego.[7]

The work of Kernberg is also helpful in understanding the antisocial disordered patient. In his view these patients have experienced savage aggression from parental relationships and often report having both observed and experienced violence in early childhood. Consequently they experience the other as potentially omnipotent and cruel. They feel that loving, mutually gratifying relationships between self and other not only can be destroyed but contain the seeds for an attack by the omnipotent other. One way to survive is by total submission. A subsequent route is to identify with the omnipotent other which gives the individual a sense of power, freedom from fear and the feeling that the only way to relate to others is by gratifying one's aggression. An alternative route is to adopt a false, cynical way of communication, totally denying the importance of relationships and becoming an innocent bystander rather than identifying with the cruel tyrant within or submitting masochistically to him. Kernberg reports that such individuals convey that they are totally convinced of the impotence of any good object relationships – the good are by definition weak and unreliable. The patient shows contempt for those who are potentially good objects. In contrast, the view is that the powerful are needed to survive but are also unreliable and invariably sadistic. The pain of having to depend upon a desperately needed but sadistic parental object is transformed into rage and expressed as rage, for the most part projected.[8]

The client group

Many of the men who find their way into the psychodrama group like George have been beaten, degraded and abandoned by one or both parents. There are too many tales of violent incest, of extreme cruelty, of children whose hands were placed on electric fires, who were fed with their own faeces or who were required to give sexual satisfaction to mothers and fathers; stories of strangers who took advantage of their vulnerable years, of children helplessly witnessing scenes of violence between parents or becoming the object of redirected anger.

Lacking in self-esteem and confidence, and angry at having being deprived as a child of what was rightfully theirs, in adult life many redirect these negative feelings onto members of society usually viewed by them as weaker. For Bowlby, treatment entails reversing these experiences in the most honest way possible.[9]

Psychodramatically this means taking the prisoner back to the primary source of his suffering by the use of 'surplus reality', which is based on Vaihinger's 'as if' principle.[10] Surplus reality transcends the limitations of reality so that the 'there and then' becomes 'the here and now' in the psychodrama enactment.

George needed to vent his anger towards his abusive father, to remove the belt from his father's hands and throw it across the room, to take his younger self in his arms and weep for what had happened to him and to question his mother's choice not to save him from his father's brutality. He also needed to understand how these repressed feelings had contributed in part to his own brutality of another, someone whom he experienced as being bullying and abusive, somewhat like his father. On the night of his crime he chose not to be a helpless victim but to attack before he was attacked. His actions went beyond self-defence and for a tragic moment the view of his victim was clouded by memory traces of a brutal father whom he had never come to terms with. 'The tendency to treat others in the same "way" as we ourselves have been treated is deep in human nature.'[11] For George to realise that he had in fact come to be like father in his treatment of the other was and has been devastating. George continues to struggle with that part of him that has taken another's life.

Psychodrama: theory and method

Psychodrama as a therapeutic method employs action methods to encourage the expression of repressed emotions and to introduce the possibility of change by correcting the maladaptive learning that has taken place. It helps the offender patient, in the context of the group, to consider in detail how his modes of procuring and dealing with significant others is influenced by his internal world and how the dysfunctional 'internal working models' he has of himself and others have been brought about by his early childhood experiences. He is encouraged to find new ways of perceiving and reacting to past and present life experiences and to understand the process by which he has come to offend.

If one is to intervene in the process whereby the offender patient redirects their repressed emotions onto others who may trigger them by their gender, position in society, attitudes, behaviour or by representing their despised weaker self, then one needs to provide an arena for these emotions to be understood by the professional and the offender. Psychodrama provides such an arena.

John, putting himself forward in a psychodrama session, said of himself: 'The police knew me as a geezer who went out and had a fight and did a bit of shoplifting and burglary, but they didn't know I would go out and rape a woman. I didn't know it myself.'

In a reconstruction of events leading up to his crime, John grabs his victim, played by a female auxiliary:

> **John**: I don't know what's going on. I don't know what's happened. I'm sorry. *(The victim lies sobbing on the floor.)* Mentally I've hurt her. I must have degraded her. We stood crying for ten minutes. I was doing more crying, I was going mental.
> **Therapist**: Show us, don't tell us.
> *(John and the auxiliary just stand crying; tears fall from John's eyes as he remembers the scene as the 'there and then' of his actions is experienced in the 'here and now' of his emotions.)*
> **John**: Every time I start thinking about what I did to you I just want to pick up a glass and smash it into my arm. I keep wishing I had lost my arm, that the doctor hadn't been able to save it [on the night of the offence he had been discharged from hospital, having cut his wrist]. It sounds crazy but I want to rip myself to bits. I hate myself for what I have done to you. The only person I wanted to hurt was my Mum. God knows what was going through my head that night, because I don't.

After the offence he walked around for two weeks sleeping in bushes in parks, drinking heavily. With the few props we have in the room we construct the symbols of a bush and ask John to roam and then settle under the bush when he is ready. He is asked to speak his thoughts out loud.

> **John**: I keep looking for excuses, but I can't find them. I say my mother's to blame but I don't know if she is. I don't know if it's just me wanting to hurt a woman for some reason. It's hard to forgive myself, it's just filthy what I've done. I did worse committing rape than my Mum ever did to me. *(John continues to roam.)* I just want to be able to trust people and love people and hold people because it must be lovely to be able to comfort somebody to say, you're all right and I like you, things like that. It must be nice.

John's mother used to cut herself in front of the children and demand that John cleared up the bucket in which she would defecate and would beat him regularly. He was left in the absence of a father to look after the young children and call the emergency services following her suicide attempts. He grew up hating his mother, wishing she were dead. In the psychodrama he was given an opportunity to speak to his mother, to role reverse with her in an attempt to come to understand her behaviour and by so doing arrive at some inner dissonance. His work finished with him placing a rose on her grave, stating that he loved and forgave her. In forgiving her in the psychodrama he was laying to rest an internal punitive mother that had led to anger and resentment that had driven him most of his life and caused him to attack not only himself but his victim.

JL Moreno developed psychodrama. Central to the understanding of psychodrama as a method of treatment is the theory of role. Moreno defined role as: 'The functioning form (role) the individual assumes in the specific moment he reacts to a specific situation in which the other person or objects are involved. The form is created by past experiences and the cultural patterns of society in which the individual lives. Every role is a fusion of private and collective elements.'[12]

It is important to remember that Moreno's existential approach would see each moment in which the individual responds as being shot through with memories of the past as well as anxieties about the present and the future.

The concept of role is usually employed to describe complexes of behaviour limited to social dimensions. Psychodrama role theory carries the concept through all dimensions of life beginning at birth and continuing through the lifetime of the individual. The total of all roles in which a person interacts is his role repertoire and it is from this complex that the personality develops. Like other role theorists, Moreno believed that the self arises out of social interaction with others. Application of psychodrama role theory requires two sets of skills: identification and intervention. In psychodrama we are concerned with the dysfunctional roles of the offender patient, his antisocial offending behaviour, and as such our first task is to identify this role and to make a role analysis. We need to observe the following aspects.

- Context of role: What is the situation or circumstances that causes our protagonist to behave in the way he does? Is it perceived rejection, humiliation etc?
- Behaviour: What does he do when presented with a set of circumstances which involves other people, and holds memory traces of his past attachment figures and earlier experiences?
- Affect: What are his feelings about the interaction?
- Cognitive distortions: What is his belief system about himself, his past, the other and the world in which he lives?
- Consequences: What is the effect on him and the other when he chooses to respond in a particular way?

Roy presented two scenes in the early part of his psychodrama, the first in the visiting room of the prison where his girlfriend boasted of her sexual exploits with other men and the second at the scene of his offence, where the prostitute he had murdered had laughed at his inability to have an erection. The context for him was similar, a situation in which a woman had left him feeling humiliated and defenceless. His behavioural response was anger. He wanted to attack his girlfriend and killed the prostitute. The belief system operating on both occasions was: women cannot be trusted; they are rejecting and aim to hurt you.

Roy was helped to see how the present situation and his offence held memory traces of past experiences, how his actions were influenced by distorted belief systems and negative feelings associated with early experiences. Roy's mother had both humiliated and hurt him emotionally as a small child. He had grown up believing that he could not trust women, that they were out to repeat his earlier experiences with his mother. Consequently women became the object of his angry feelings.

It was important for Roy to return to the scene of childhood to address his mother, but in a way it was not possible for him to do so then. In the psychodrama he became angry and tearful. It was equally important for him to understand his own actions arising out of distorted cognitions and motivations. Roy needed to differentiate between anger at mother from present anger at other and self for maintaining belief systems developed in the past and transferred onto his victim. 'Self criticism of one's own actions can only follow if these actions are accessible or reportable.'[13] Psychodrama provides an arena for this to happen by the use of such techniques as mirroring, doubling and concretisation. As the psychodrama came to its conclusion, Roy knelt down by his victim, having understood his own process by which he had come to kill her. He acknowledged his actions and how she had become an innocent victim of his own unresolved issues and begged her forgiveness. Sadly too late for his victim, but when he returned to the scene with his girlfriend he brought together both the affective and cognitive elements of the enactment sequence in order to integrate the work that had taken place and explored new ways of dealing with the situation. This element of the psychodrama is known as role training.

A classical psychodrama consists of three stages: the warm-up, the enactment and the sharing.

The warm-up stage

Each session starts with the warm-up, which increases a sense of trust and builds group cohesion through techniques that encourage interactions between group members. It stimulates the spontaneity of group members and helps focus on personal issues. Other group members who resonate with the issues presented select the offender patient whose work will be the focus of the enactment. In this way the selected protagonist works for the group, carrying the group's concerns, as well as for himself. In the enactment stage the offender patient with the support of group members and the therapist explores the issues heightened by the warm-up process.

The enactment stage

In psychodrama there is no script; the drama is spontaneous, created in the moment by the protagonist, group members and the therapist. Because psychodrama is intrinsically an action method the protagonist is encouraged to move quickly into action, creating the space in which events took place and an experience of re-experiencing rather than retelling. The physical setting of scenes and their portrayal evokes memories associated with the space and counters the distortions and evasive manoeuvres that may be introduced by verbal disclosure.[14]

The characters the offender patient places on the psychodrama stage are part of his internal world. The choice of certain group members to play these parts, auxiliary egos, are determined by complex factors which Moreno, the creator of the method, defines as 'tele', the two-way flow between people.[15] I suggest they are also determined by transference reactions towards other group members.

Playing the role of an auxiliary ego can in itself be therapeutic, often providing the offender patient with an opportunity to develop other ways of being not hitherto experienced or to discover aspects of himself that he has chosen to deny. Jim, having been selected to hold the role of the good father in a psychodrama, is required to tell a fairy tale to the protagonist. After the psychodrama he shares that he himself has a son with whom he has little contact and vows to read to him on his release from prison. Ricky, an armed robber, is asked to hold the role of a rapist. Returning after the session, he is distressed and disturbed. 'I realise that I used my gun in the same way as Andy used his penis. I always thought that sex offenders were the lowest of the low, scum, but really there is no difference between us.'

The process of holding the role of an other also helps to develop some understanding and empathy for the other's position: 'Playing George's Mum made me think of how it must have been like for my Mum'. 'Being George's victim made me think of how it was for my victim' is not an uncommon comment.

The sharing stage

The final section of the psychodrama is the sharing. During this time other group members come together to share what they resonate with in the psychodrama that has taken place. It might be that through the session they themselves have been in tears or have found it difficult to contain their own anger. They may have come up and doubled for the protagonist, a technique whereby a group member expresses thoughts and feeling that the protagonist is finding difficult to express. In Roy's psychodrama, as he faced a terrifying mother at the age of four he could only sit and weep in the space provided. Someone from the group got up and sat beside him and voiced his anger. He knew something of this mother and identified with the young child. In the sharing stage he spoke of his own rejecting mother and his own anger towards her and how he had displaced these unresolved feelings onto others.

Others may have not been actively involved in holding roles but somehow the story, though different, holds some similarities to their own life. Martin, who prided himself in keeping a body book of 300 bodies that he had killed as a professional mercenary, was unable to have any feelings for what he had done or for anything or anyone. He wore heavy-rimmed spectacles that shielded his eyes from conveying any sign of emotion. In his own psychodrama he had been very much in control, simply going through the process of attempting to understand why he was so cut off from his emotions. Several sessions later as he watched another group member kneel remorsefully by the side of his now dead mother whom he had mocked for looking so ugly (he had gone into the bathroom and seen how her body had been ravaged by a mastectomy) Martin began to sob, so loudly that we had to halt the action and ask another member to offer a comforting and containing arm. In the sharing he said he realised that the last time he had cried was when his mother had died. He remembered after her death he had come into the house crying, having got into a fight with other boys in the street. His father attacked him for his weakness and told him to get back on the street and not come in until he had won the fight. 'I have never cried since that day.' In watching his colleague's work he had accessed his own grief at losing his mother and reconnected with all that she had stood for and from which he had distanced himself by over-identifying with the internalised abusive father. Several months later as I bumped into him in open conditions he smiled and asked, 'Do you like my glasses? I don't need to hide anymore – thanks.' He was wearing rimless spectacles.

There is an ordered simplicity in the psychodrama process. In working with the protagonist we:

- begin with the present problem
- find similarities in the recent past
- discover the linkages to the deep past
- help the client understand his process in life
- achieve a catharsis, if necessary
- concretise the issues, choices and actions that keep the client in the present dysfunctional state
- help him see the options in life
- aid in the integration of the cognitive and the affective
- achieve closure and healing so that the client can carry out in life what has been learned in therapy.[16]

Most psychotherapeutic processes rely on the therapeutic relationship to represent symbolically the client's internal world. Kernberg emphasises the difficulty and danger of this approach when working with a client group who have dangerous and violent inherent paranoid transference reactions.

Psychodrama is also concerned with the client's symbolic representation of his external and internal reality world, but the representation follows a different route through the enactment itself, relying on auxiliaries and scene setting to represent time and place. Psychodrama lays fantasy out in three dimensions and relieves the therapist of the task of becoming everything to the protagonist and the recipient of his primitive rage.

Dave was referred to the psychodrama programme for his violent paranoid behaviour. He would often talk about going into a black hole where he lost touch with all reality. 'My fear is that if I go there and mistake you for my mother you could be dead.' Dave's mother had suffered from severe schizophrenia and had played with his emotions unmercifully. Sometimes she would be loving and caring, at other times she would chase him around the table with a carving knife. I had the potential of becoming his manipulating, untrustworthy mother who, in the midst of his emotional vulnerability, would cast my blow. Choosing not to work with his transference reactions, we agreed that he would ask for clarification or share with me and the group when he perceived my actions to be manipulative or potentially harmful or felt on the edge of his black hole. In this way I became a little less like the mother and he less like the helpless son. When it came to a point when he had to face his mother in the psychodrama, represented by an empty chair, and he faced his 'black hole', I was able to stand alongside as director and facilitator rather than someone who was perceived as out to play mind games.

There are inevitably difficulties in this approach; the fact that offender patients, particularly those of a violent nature, often fear their emotional side means that 'If I lose control, what then?' is a familiar question. Experiencing emotions that have not been dealt with raises anxiety as to whether the group, the protagonist and the therapist can survive the emotions that need expression. There needs to be an atmosphere of tolerance and acceptance. Such hostile statements from other prisoners as 'I have no time for sex offenders; you are animals; I feel intimidated by your violence' fail to provide a setting that encourages the offender to explore those shameful aspects of themselves. When Bill held in his arms the son he had murdered, a hostile comment could have forced him back into a world of isolation and defensive manoeuvres, leaving him unable to confront the unspeakable.

The group's readiness to deal with certain issues is paramount to the work. It is inadvisable to go ahead if the group is not warmed up to the protagonist and to the issues and to itself. It is essential to realise the group's need for containment.

Early in a session as the group were beginning to know each other and find out why they had elected to come onto psychodrama, Ed declared that he was impatient to start work. Knowing a little about the method, he turned to the group and stated: 'I wouldn't be the one who has to play my uncle who sexually abused me at my father's grave.' The members physically retreated into silence, knowing a little of the anger Ed held towards this abusive uncle. Ed was ready to begin work, but neither the group or myself was. It was some six months before we could undertake this work; before the group felt safe enough and I felt safe enough with the group to begin to understand how this suppressed anger had impacted on Ed's life and to allow him the space to confront both his abusive uncle and his abusive self. When we did, a mattress from one of the cells protected the auxiliary who offered to take on the role and Ed used his filled laundry bag and was directed to confine his rage to the mattress. As often happens, behind the rage were tears of hurt and sadness for what had happened to him as a child. The good father, who had not been able to protect him at the time, in the psychodrama came to his rescue and offered comfort and so the internal abusive figure that Ed had identified with was replaced by a more benign but proactive role.

'What are you going to get if you put me in a cage and pump me with a stick? You are going to get me worse than I came in. I know about that. But show me love and care – I don't know about that, that's difficult, that does your head in.' The words of a prisoner who took part in a BBC Actuality programme on psychodrama at Grendon. By caring, we tackle these internal figures and the associated emotions that remain alive and active. I would cautiously suggest that psychodrama provides the notion of 'maternal containment' described by Bion, in that it manages the internal rage associated with these internal figures and transforms it into some something more manageable which can be integrated into the ego. In addition, it helps the offender patient to develop trust in themselves and in relationships.

References

1   Holmes J (1993) Attachment theory: a biological basis for psychotherapy? *British Journal of Psychiatry.* **163**: 430–8.
2   Heard D and Lake B (1986) The attachment dynamic in adult life. *British Journal of Psychiatry.* **149**: 430–8.
3   Henderson A (1974) Care eliciting behaviour in man. *Journal of Nervous and Mental Diseases.* **159**: 172–81.
4   Rodeheffer M (1979) quoted in J Bowlby *Making and Breaking of Affectional Bonds.* Tavistock, London.
5   Bowlby J (1979) *Making and Breaking of Affectional Bonds.* Tavistock, London.
6   Bion WR (1970) *Attention and Interpretation.* Tavistock, London.
7   Winnicott DW (1965) *The Maturational Process and the Facilitating Environment.* Hogarth Press, London.
8   Kernberg O (1984) *Severe Personality Disorder: psychotherapeutic strategies.* Yale University Press, New Haven and London.
9   Bowlby J (1979) *Making and Breaking of Affectional Bonds.* Tavistock, London.
10 Vaihinger H (1911) *Philosophie des Als Ob.* Reutner & Reinhard, Berlin (English translation: *The Philosophy of As If*).
11 Bowlby J (1998) *A Secure Base – clinical applications of attachment theory.* Routledge, London.
12 Fox J (1987) *The Essential Moreno.* Springer, New York.
13 Sarbin T and Allen V (1968) Role theory. In: G Lindzey and E Aronson (eds) *The Handbook of Social Psychology Vol. 1.* Addison Wesley, Reading, MA.
14 Meloy J (1998) *The Psychopathic Mind.* Aronsona Inc., London.
15 Moreno JL (1975) *Psychodrama Volume 2.* Beacon House, New York.
16 Goldman E and Morrison D (1984) *Psychodrama Experience and Process.* Kendall/Hunt Pub. Co., Dubugue, Iowa.

Chapter 14

After life imprisonment: the role of the probation service

Catherine Appleton

The number of life-sentenced offenders has increased significantly in recent years and the lifer population across England and Wales is now in excess of 5000 offenders. Under the current system, lifers are released on licence to probation areas in the community '. . . whose responsibility it is to contribute to public protection through the supervision of life-sentenced offenders'.[1] The life sentence provides the power to recall offenders to prison at any time for the remainder of his or her life as a result of unacceptable behaviour, the commission of an offence or other breaches of the life licence.[2,3] The release and resettlement of life-sentenced offenders therefore poses a critical challenge to criminal justice professionals: the challenge of ensuring the public is protected from dangerous offenders, whilst simultaneously protecting the rights of individuals.

This chapter arises from research carried out by myself and colleagues at the Centre for Criminological Research and Probation Studies Unit, University of Oxford, investigating the role of the Probation Service in the resettlement process of discretionary life-sentenced offenders.[4] Discretionary lifers represent a substantial minority of the overall life-sentenced population. On 28 February 2003, there were 1683 prisoners serving discretionary life sentences.[5] This represented 31% of the total life-sentenced population of 5352 prisoners; the remainder were serving mandatory life sentences for murder. A life sentence is mandatory for persons convicted of murder and automatic for those sentenced for a second serious sexual or violent offence which carries a life sentence (Section 2).[6] A life sentence is discretionary for a number of other serious offences, including attempted murder, manslaughter, rape, armed robbery, arson, criminal damage with intent to endanger life and some drug offences. Discretionary life sentences can only be imposed when: the offence is considered grave enough to require a very long sentence; the offender is a person of mental instability who, if at liberty, presents a grave danger to the public; it appears that the offender will remain unstable and a potential danger for a long or uncertain time.[7,8]

The law relating to discretionary lifers significantly changed in 1991 following a decision of the European Court of Human Rights in *Thynne, Wilson and Gunnell v United Kingdom*. The decision established the right of those subject to a discretionary life sentence to regular and independent review once the 'tariff' (punishment) period of their sentence had ended. Discretionary Lifer Panels (DLPs) of the Parole Board were subsequently introduced in 1992 as an independent body with the status of a court and the power to review the lawfulness of continued detention beyond the tariff. DLPs were given the responsibility by Parliament to direct the Home Secretary to release a life-sentenced prisoner only if they are '. . . satisfied that it is no longer necessary for the protection of the public that the prisoner should be confined' (Section 28 (6)).[6] Once this condition has been fulfilled, discretionary lifers are released on life licence to the National Probation Service which has the responsibility to safeguard the public through the process of supervision, and the authority to recall life-sentenced offenders to custody at any time for any breach of the life licence. The effective supervision and management of lifers is therefore fundamental to the process of resettlement.

By drawing upon empirical research, this chapter attempts to provide insights into the process of supervising discretionary life-sentenced offenders, and the factors which enhance resettlement. Following this introduction, the chapter contains four main sections: the first section briefly describes the research methodology of the study; section two summarises the characteristics of the sample of discretionary life-sentenced offenders; the third section examines the overall process of supervising discretionary lifers; and the final section highlights some of the implications of the study.

Research methodology

The research was commissioned by the Home Office, as part of its *Dangerous People with Severe Personality Disorder Initiative*,[9] to investigate the role of the Probation Service following the release of discretionary life-sentenced offenders. The main aims of the research were: to identify the factors involved in supervision; to improve understanding of the individual risk factors associated with discretionary life-sentenced offenders; and to assist the Probation Service in improving the prospect of successful resettlement. The research was carried out between June 2002 and September 2003 and the main methods employed were: semi-structured interviews with probation practitioners; content analysis of offenders' probation files; collection of documentation and statistical information from the Parole Board; and observation of a number of DLP hearings.

A sample of 138 discretionary life-sentenced offenders was provided by the Parole Board at the start of the project, all of whom had been released from prison during the first five years of the DLP process (1992–1997). For a variety of reasons, it was not possible to collect full data on every offender and, in total, 113 probation officer interviews were carried out and 117 probation files were analysed across probation areas in England and Wales.

Offender characteristics

Using data collected from the Parole Board and probation files, this section summarises some of the key characteristics of the sample of discretionary lifers.

Demographic data

Of the overall sample population, 96% were male and, where ethnicity was known, 94% were white. In August 2003, the mean age of the offenders was 54 years, and 50% were aged between 45 and 60 years. At the time of the fieldwork, 18 (13%) of the offenders in the sample population had died, 14 in the community and 4 in prison. Data gathered from probation files revealed that almost a third (30%) of the sample had been placed in local authority care during childhood, 26% had attended an approved school and just over a fifth (22%) had experienced another form of institutional care (such as time spent in borstal institutions). The majority of the sample population (63%) had experienced some form of physical, sexual or emotional abuse during childhood.

Criminal history and index offence

At the time of the life sentence, 87% of this offender population had previous convictions, with an average of 17 convictions. The age at first criminal conviction ranged from 8 to 56 years, and the mean age at first conviction was 19. Not surprisingly, those with the largest numbers of previous convictions were also more likely to have been first convicted at a younger age.[10]

The index offence for almost half the sample was homicide (49%); 22% received a life sentence for sexual offences; 14% had committed other violent offences and 4% of the sample were arsonists. Over a third (35%) of all the index offences, for which offenders were convicted, contained a sexual element. Probation file data revealed that all the homicide offenders were convicted of manslaughter on the grounds of diminished responsibility under the *Homicide Act 1957*. Sexual offences included rape, repeat sex offences, buggery, indecent assault and unlawful sexual intercourse. The 'other violence' category included offences such as attempted murder, grievous bodily harm with intent and wounding with intent to commit grievous bodily harm. The arson offenders were usually repeat arsonists or those who had committed arson with intent to endanger life.

Release status

Given that life-sentenced offenders, following their release from prison, can be recalled at any time under Section 39 of the *Criminal Justice Act 1991*, the 'release status' for offenders in the sample inevitably fluctuated.[2] While there were 12 offenders for whom the release status was not known, at the time of the fieldwork 65% of the total sample were released, of whom three-quarters were under supervision, 9% had had the supervision requirement lifted and 16% had died on licence. A quarter of offenders (26%) were recalled, 3% of whom had subsequently died in custody. However, probation file data revealed that one third of offenders (32%) in the sample had been released during the life sentence more than once and some of the releases and recalls had occurred prior to the establishment of the DLP process. For example, one offender had been released from prison five times in total, over an 18-year period, only one of which had been a DLP release in 1994.

For the purpose of analysis, the introduction of the DLP process in 1992 was taken as a baseline and, by August 2003, 54 out of 117 offenders had been recalled at least once (46%). The majority of these (59%) had been recalled for behaviour that gave rise to concern, such as failure to comply with licence conditions. The remainder were recalled either for a reconviction (20%) or both a reconviction and behaviour that gave rise to concern (20%). Of those reconvicted, 11 were recalled for sexual offences, 6 for violent offences, 2 were recalled for robbery offences and 3 for other offences. In three cases the recall offence was serious enough to warrant a second discretionary life sentence.

Over a third (37%) of the offenders who had been recalled once since 1992 had been re-released and were living in the community. There were 9 offenders (17% of all those recalled) who had been released twice and had been recalled to custody. For all recalled cases, the minimum time spent in the community prior to the offenders' most recent recall date was four days and the maximum time period was almost nine years, with the mean length of time in the community being close to three years. In comparison, the offenders released into the community via a DLP hearing who had never been recalled spent a minimum of just over four years in the community and a maximum of 10 years, with an average length of time of just over eight years.

Mental health

In the case of *R v Wilkinson* (1983), Lord Lane Chief Justice explained that:

> 'With few exceptions [the discretionary life sentence] . . . is reserved, broadly speaking, for offenders who for one reason or another cannot be dealt with under the Mental Health Act, yet who are in a mental state which makes them dangerous to the life or limb of members of the public.'

It was therefore not surprising to find that the vast majority (97%) of offenders in the sample displayed mental instability at the time of the life sentence. Indeed, 82% of the offenders had previously been diagnosed with more than one mental health problem, and 50% of the sample had between two and five mental health concerns. For example, almost three-quarters of the offenders (74%) had displayed a pattern of impulsive behaviour; 61% had experienced difficulties coping; 39% were diagnosed with psychiatric problems; a fifth of the sample had attempted suicide and a quarter of the offenders had other mental health problems, such as gross emotional immaturity or deviant sexual fantasies. To some extent, the mental health problems of these offenders had been exacerbated by substance abuse; 60% were assessed as having alcohol problems and almost a quarter (23%) had drug problems.

At the time of the study, data from the Hare Psychopathy Checklist[11,12,13] were available on 106 offenders. According to Hare,[11] the characteristics of psychopaths are as follows:

> 'Interpersonally, psychopaths are grandiose, egocentric, manipulative, dominant, forceful, and cold hearted. . . . Behaviourally, psychopaths are impulsive and sensation seeking and they readily violate social norms. The most obvious expressions of these predispositions involve criminality, substance abuse and failure to fulfil social obligations and responsibilities.'

Hare's Psychopathy Checklist (PCL-R) consists of a 20-item checklist to be scored on the basis of collateral file information and a semi-structured clinical interview. The PCL-R produces a score between 0 and 40; the higher the score, the more psychopathic the individual. Sixty-eight per cent of the offenders in the sample scored 25 or more on the PCL-R, indicating a significant level of psychopathy in a UK-based sample.[14] The next section of this chapter highlights some of the problems faced by probation practitioners in attempting to supervise and manage effectively the risk of these offenders in the community.

Supervising lifers

A convenient reference point for practitioners supervising lifers is the Prison Service *Lifer Manual*, which states that:

> 'The life sentence prisoner will have regular contact with the Probation Service throughout his or her period in prison from remand to release and whilst under supervision in the community on life licence.'[15]

This section attempts to summarise some of the main characteristics of lifer supervision from case allocation through to the training of practitioners. Practitioner interviews and data from probation files help illuminate work at the front-line with serious offenders.

Allocation

The Lifer Manual states that the supervising officer should be an

> '. . . experienced practitioner who must be able to cope with the pressures and anxieties of this kind of work'.[15]

Of those interviewed, the majority of probation officers (60%) were experienced supervisors and had supervised three or more life-sentenced offenders. For a fifth (19%) of officers the current supervisee was their first lifer case, but they had been probation officers for more than two years prior to the start of the supervision process. While the majority of interviewees were experienced officers, the allocation process varied considerably between each probation area, as exemplified in the following remarks:

> 'It was quite random. I saw him once as a duty officer on his release and we seemed to get on, plus I think he was previously allocated to a black female officer and had a slightly racist streak in him – therefore he came to me (white male officer).'

> 'It was because he was released to my patch – coverage was organised on a geographical basis.'

> 'It may have been that I'm an experienced PO, but I think they were basically scrabbling for people.'

All of those interviewed agreed, however, that contact with life-sentenced offenders should be regarded as different from other types of supervision, particularly because of the gravity of the offence and the long-term nature of supervision. One practitioner commented that lifer supervision:

> '. . . is a specialist area which is not given the attention it deserves. I think there's a need for increased resources and training for experienced staff to work with high risk offenders. At the moment there are few incentives to encourage staff to work in this field with more credit being given to other aspects.'

The Lifer Manual also specifies a pairing system:

> 'Arrangements must also be made for a contact with a second officer familiar with the case whom the supervising officer can consult whenever difficulties arise and, particularly, to take over supervision of the licensee during the absence of the designated supervising probation officer.'[15]

Probation officers generally supported this approach; it was accepted as good practice in the supervision of lifers and, in some areas, a 'back up officer' was in place for work with lifers. However, due to limited resources and large caseloads, there was little evidence of this policy in practice and there was scope for clearer support structures to be in place. As one officer commented: 'We should have a paired worker, but if I do not have time to read the file, how will a pair be able to do this?'

There were several officers who commented on the weight of responsibility of supervising lifers and the fear of the consequences of 'something going wrong', despite the management of such offenders being the responsibility of the probation area as a whole. For example, in one case an offender had been supervised for five years by an officer, and was recalled in 2000 for a serious sexual offence and received a second discretionary life sentence. The supervisor stated:

> 'I feel for the victims of his latest offences and I feel that I've failed the case and the Service. With hindsight, my supervision relied too much on the offender's feedback. Back-up support only came in when things went wrong.'

Continuity of contact

Previous research suggests that long-term prisoners seek '. . . some kind of personal relationship and rapport with probation officers' and that the relationship is readily enhanced if officers are able to demonstrate '. . . consistency and reliability, courtesy, honest, directness [and] knowledge of the system'.[16] Across the probation areas, there were only a few areas where it was local policy for officers to retain lifer cases when they moved posts within a county. However, almost all interviewees (93%) emphasised the importance of the continuity of officer in lifer supervision, providing that support networks for officers were firmly in place in order to avoid complacency or collusive relationships. Practitioners cited the 'need to have a rapport' with lifers in order to build an open and trusting relationship due to the complex and indeterminate nature of risk assessment. One officer emphasised:

> 'We still need to establish relationships if we are to work with difficult people. There is a danger of passing people around in that no-one ever gets to know a lifer at all – they will not engage in the process.'

Risk assessment

The supervision of discretionary life-sentenced offenders is centrally concerned with the management of risk due to the nature and gravity of the offence committed. Over the past decade, the Probation Service has become increasingly concerned with public protection and developing risk assessment policies and strategies for managing dangerous offenders. Practitioners overwhelmingly agreed that the frequency and purpose of contact should be determined by the level of risk and it was clear from file data that supervision contact increased when probation officers had concerns about an individual. Kemshall argues for 'defensible' rather than 'defensive' decisions.

Defensive practice is dependent on the precautionary principle which focuses on 'worst case' scenarios and low tolerance of errors, whereas defensible decision-making occurs when '. . . reliable assessment methods have been used, information is collected and thoroughly evaluated, decisions are recorded, staff work within agency policies and procedures and staff communicate with others and seek information they do not have'.[17] While officers were clearly aware of the importance of risk assessment and management in the supervision process, there were sometimes obstacles to achieving this:

> 'The main feeling is that caseloads need to come down. Large caseloads do not take into account the type of people we're supervising. There is a need to look specifically at the work of resettlement officers and enable proper risk assessment, proper planning and proper release plans. Otherwise it sets everyone up to fail – we are all vulnerable so that we are ultra cautious – we do not have time to make defensible decisions. Risk assessment is risky – you need

all the facts. I feel we are being forced into positions of making decisions on inadequate information.'

There were, however, some notable examples of a joined-up approach to resettlement, focusing on the continuous management of risk and sharing the responsibility of decision-making. For example, in some cases, close working relationships between probation and mental health services had developed as a result of the contact made through life licence conditions. As one officer illustrated:

'He is low risk at the moment so there are longer gaps in supervision, but he sees the psychiatric social worker fortnightly and psychiatrist bi-monthly as part of his licence. We also meet as a group with the offender once every six months. This means I can discuss any decisions to be made and the responsibility is shared. This has had a very positive impact – has helped him resettle.'

The recent development of *Multi Agency Public Protection Arrangements*[18,19] was seen across probation areas to have a paramount role in determining the best local response to the issue of risk management and was commonly described as a 'vast improvement to supervision'. Practitioners expressed confidence that these strategies provided a good opportunity to ensure that high-risk offenders in contact with probation were managed through a coordinated, multi-agency approach to risk assessment and management, within which 'defensible decisions can be reached'.

Management oversight and Lifer Unit liaison

More than three-quarters of interviewees (77%) stated that they had enough support from middle and senior managers, but the amount of involvement in lifer cases by managers varied considerably. Much contact between managers and officers to discuss lifer cases was close and supportive:

'My SPO carries out monthly supervision – very supportive, an excellent line manager – the ACPO signs quarterly reports and comments where appropriate and the CPO has put the appropriate policies in place, plus there's a great deal of informal support within the office and with my co-worker for this case.'

Support was not always good, however, and sometimes senior officers were described as distant and dismissive:

'The management view that "lifers equal no work" should be changed, particularly when they are in an institution or if they have been out for a year. This is what the officers are being told by the management. I wish the Service and the Home Office would give more priority to lifer work. Resettling people in the community is not cheap.'

This view has been shared by HM Inspectorates of Prison and Probation:

> 'The importance of work with lifers must be acknowledged due to the gravity of the offences, the lifelong consequences for victims and families, the indeterminate nature of the sentence and the sense of responsibility experienced by staff working with them.'[1]

It therefore follows that probation management should give greater recognition to the supervision of lifers, and guidance should be in place across all probation areas to ensure clear support networks for probation officers undertaking this type of supervision.

Probation officers supervising lifers are required to provide reports to the Home Office Lifer Unit, both to report progress and flag up any difficulties. The research findings revealed that arrangements between the Lifer Unit and probation areas were seen as limited in relation to routine reporting, but effective in a crisis situation: 'They are very quick to respond on the issue of a warning letter or recall . . . much quicker than responding to a request to cancel supervision.' The Lifer Manual[15] states that consideration can be given to cancelling the supervision element of the life licence after a minimum of four years; although for sex offenders cancellation will not be considered until 10 years have elapsed. Interview and file data confirmed that there were a few cases in which officers had applied for the supervision requirement to be lifted and had received an inadequate response. In a few instances licensees continued to be supervised for no apparently valid reason, where the offender concerned appeared to be personally, socially and economically settled. While interviewees acknowledged that the Lifer Unit needs to 'err on the side of caution' with a presumption in favour of public protection, this should be balanced with a presumption in favour of release from supervision when the suspension of supervision is assessed to be safe.

Training of supervisors

Over three-quarters of officers interviewed (82%) stated a need for training in the supervision of discretionary lifers. The following comment made by one of the interviewees sums up some of the issues raised:

> 'There's a colossal need for lifer training – it's a huge gap! What tends to happen is after three or four years you find you're allocated a lifer – you're seen to be capable – but the requirements are found out by accident. Seniors are not necessarily trained either. You learn on the hoof. Going to the Lifer Unit would be helpful. We need training in risk assessment and what the Lifer Unit are really looking for.'

There was considerable demand for training courses on the overall process of the lifer system, from the pre-sentence stage through to oral hearings and community supervision:

> '. . . lifers often know more than the officers, as they know their system. It would be useful to have an A–Z breakdown of what you have to cover and where things slot into place.'

Indeed, the Lifer Manual was regarded as a convenient reference point, but insufficiently detailed with regard to the complexity of issues (some probation areas had produced their own supplemental guidance). Consideration should also be given as to how to prepare probation officers before they first undertake supervision of a life-sentenced offender. It was with concern that one officer stated:

> 'With the allocation of lifers, you're often thrown in at the deep end – [It is a case of] "Who hasn't had a lifer?" – You basically learn on the job and ask your colleagues . . . but you shouldn't get a lifer until you're properly trained in risk assessment and know the prison system and how lifers differ.'

It may be the case that lifer supervision is inherently problematic in that there are relatively few cases and yet the work is sufficiently technical and challenging to warrant specialist knowledge, skills and training. However, given the gravity of the life sentence and the high level of responsibility in managing the risk of life-sentenced offenders, it is clear that sufficient opportunity should be provided for practitioners and managers to gain the necessary skills and knowledge of the lifer system.

Resettlement and recall

At the time of the fieldwork, 81 probation officers were supervising lifers in the community and 32 were supervising those recalled. Officers were asked to identify problems that had occurred for each offender during the licence period and discuss how these had been addressed during supervision. The most common problem to be addressed in supervision during the resettlement period was mental health (49%). This was followed by personal relationships (45%), employment (42%), alcohol and drug issues (35%), accommodation (35%), other problems, such as physical health and institutionalisation (33%), family relationships (31%), financial difficulties (27%) and criminal peers (11%).

Through the Prison Gate,[20] a joint Prison and Probation Inspectorates thematic review of through-care, provides a challenging definition of resettlement as:

> 'A systematic and evidence-based process by which actions are taken to work with the offender in custody and on release, so that communities are better protected from harm and reoffending is significantly reduced. It encompasses the totality of work with prisoners, their families and significant others in partnership with statutory and voluntary agencies.'

The review also goes on to suggest that there has been insufficient focus on the 'basics of resettlement', such as finance, accommodation, relationships, employment and drug and alcohol problems, and that attention to those areas is vital if resettlement is to be achieved successfully. All offenders in the sample population had faced more than one problem following their release from custody and there was clearly a need for the engagement of a number of agencies. As one probation officer stated: 'Getting a job is the main goal, but unless his accommodation and alcohol problems are dealt with, any form of employment is highly unlikely'. While space does not permit a full analysis of each of the problem areas, mental health, the most common risk factor, is discussed below.

The sample exhibited a wide range of mental illnesses, including depression, anxiety, schizophrenia and agoraphobia. The vast majority of those with mental health problems had experienced 'bouts of depression' at some stage following release. The main way in which mental health problems were addressed during the licence period was via referral to psychiatric or psychological interventions, although this was usually complemented by one-to-one work during supervision sessions. In addition, some probation officers had benefited from a joined-up approach to the assessment and management of mental health difficulties, and the majority were optimistic about the development of Public Protection Arrangements.[17,18] In one case, the supervision requirement of the licence had been lifted, but psychiatric oversight remained and was seen as critical to the offender's successful resettlement.

However, there were a few cases for which mental health care was lacking and offenders had experienced difficulties coping with life outside prison. Interviewees observed that inter-agency coordination in the assessment and management of mental health problems was vital. For example, after being released to a probation hostel, one female offender, who had been diagnosed with schizophrenia at the time of the offence, returned voluntarily to custody as she was 'in need of a sanctuary' and 'unable to cope with life outside' due to a lack of adequate mental health care provision in the community.

File and interview data also highlighted the problem of psychopathic disorder. In a number of cases there had been a psychiatric assessment stating that the offender was '. . . a psychopath and therefore untreatable'. In such cases, interviewees frequently noted that while there was no diagnosed mental health problem, there were clearly mental health issues that needed to be addressed during supervision. Some probation officers pointed to a 'brick wall' of mental health support due to a reluctance to support this admittedly very difficult group of offenders. Understanding and managing psychopathic disorder was a key issue highlighted by many probation officers and there was scope for further training and support. In one case, the offender was released to a psychiatric hospital and recalled back to prison after only two months in the community. After interviewing the supervisor and reading the file data, the research interviewer commented:

'There was a consistent view from psychiatrists that he did not have a mental health illness and he was diagnosed with a personality disorder. It was probably inevitable that he would not be seen as acceptable to psychiatric services and social services were not keen to have him in their area. The supervisor was on holiday at the time and recall was seen as the easiest option for all concerned. It was clear that release was not properly planned and the supervisor felt the offender had been "set up to fail". The offender has now been in prison for 22 years – apart from a small outing in 1993.'

Indeed, there were a small number of worrying cases which had been released for a short period of time in the community, but had subsequently been recalled to closed conditions, and appeared to probation officers to be 'stuck in the system' due to the difficulties encountered during resettlement. As Hood and Shute[21] observed in an unpublished study on Parole Board decisions reviewing life sentence prisoners:

> 'The problem is that once [prisoners] have been identified as difficult or recalcitrant cases they have been so long in the system that no one knows how to plan a risk-free resettlement.'

Risk of recall

The life sentence provides the power to recall the offender to prison for the remainder of his or her natural life (Section 39).[2] Recall to prison is both a preventative measure and a penalty, with the public interest as its central objective. The decision to recall is a collective decision of the probation officer, senior probation management, the Home Office and the Parole Board based on the offender's behaviour. This is especially so when recall is used because the behaviour causes concern and fear for public safety as opposed to the commission of a further offence. Recall is a sanction of considerable gravity since the offender has to return to custody for an indefinite period of time. Coker and Martin observed that to request an offender's recall is an exercise of power requiring one of the most difficult professional judgements that a probation officer has to make.[22]

As identified earlier in this chapter, just under half (46%) of the sample were recalled following the introduction of the DLP process in 1992, some of whom had been re-released or re-recalled. There are a number of different measures that could be used to determine the 'success' or 'failure' of releasing offenders on life licence. Given the number of recalls experienced by the offenders and the differing reasons leading to a recall, attempting to classify successes and failures in the sample was a difficult task. Using a crude definition that successful cases were those offenders who had not been recalled since the introduction of the DLP process in 1992 and failures were offenders who had been recalled, it was possible to investigate which factors were significantly associated with recall.

The following characteristics, in order of significance, were associated with a higher risk of recall:

1　misusing alcohol following release
2　having been 18 years or younger at the time of first conviction
3　having a higher number of previous convictions
4　scoring 25 or more on Hare's psychopathy checklist
5　not having psychological problems at the time of the offence
6　being sexually motivated at the time of the offence
7　not knowing the victim

8 having been abused during childhood
9 having committed an index offence which included a sexual element
10 having experienced local authority care during childhood
11 having used alcohol as a disinhibitor for the index offence
12 having been hostile to the home probation officer during custody
13 having mental health problems following release.

While it was difficult to quantify the level and standard of probation supervision before and after release from custody, the analysis suggested that lifers who received extensive contact during the custodial period were less likely to be recalled, although this was not a statistically significant relationship.

Conclusion

Probation supervision has always been an activity with competing requirements; concern for the welfare of offenders rests alongside the need to ensure enforcement of the law and to protect the public. The supervision and management of high risk offenders has provided a major challenge to the Probation Service in recent years, particularly when that work has had to be completed under the watchful eye of the media. It should be noted however that effective practice with lifers begins with the core social work skill – building open and trusting relationships. Training and development opportunities in lifer supervision for both managers and practitioners are essential, and given the gravity of offences and indeterminate nature of supervision, front-line staff should be able to expect a significant degree of managerial support in order to equip them for the difficult task of reintegrating an extremely socially excluded group of offenders.

The research outlined above suggests that resettling lifers demands the engagement of a large number of agencies. Creating a holistic approach and ensuring agencies give sufficient priority at a local level is essential. Indeed, where a structured, joined-up approach to addressing problems was in place, practitioners felt better able to make accurate risk assessments and were more confident that resettlement difficulties were being addressed. The research also found that one of the central characteristics of the supervision and risk management of discretionary lifers should be the promotion of defensible decision-making. In a review of the work of Public Protection Panels, Maguire et al.[18] have observed that such an approach '. . . offers the best chance of simultaneously providing effective protection to the public, safeguarding the rights of offenders, and protecting decision makers from unfair recriminations when new crimes are committed despite their best efforts'.

While this chapter has covered a range of issues, much more could be said about the task of supervising lifers. The main limitation of the research is the lack of information from the offenders themselves. Further research is needed if we are to understand how offenders themselves interpret and respond to the various attempts to help them, and how these have impacted on their own personal efforts to resettle after life imprisonment.

Acknowledgements

Thanks are due to Ros Burnett and Aidan Wilcox for their helpful comments on an earlier draft of this chapter. The research that this chapter is based on could not have been possible without the help and support of a large number of people. In particular, grateful thanks go to Colin Roberts, Ann Barker, Jenny Roberts, the highly skilled research interviewers, colleagues at the Home Office, and to the probation officers themselves who talked openly about their experiences. Thanks are also due to David Jones for his editorial assistance and patience.

References

1　Her Majesty's Inspectorates of Prisons and Probation (1999) *Lifers: A Joint Thematic Review*. Home Office, London.
2　Great Britain (1991) *Criminal Justice Act 1991*. Home Office, London.
3　JUSTICE (1996) *Sentenced for Life: reform of the law and procedure for those sentenced to life imprisonment*. JUSTICE, London.
4　Appleton C and Roberts C (2003) *The Resettlement of Discretionary Life-sentenced Offenders*. Unpublished report to the Home Office.
5　Hollis V and Goodman M (2003) *Prison Population Brief, England and Wales*. Home Office, London.
6　Great Britain (1997) *Crime (Sentences) Act 1997*. Stationery Office, London.
7　*R v Hodgson* (1967) 52 Cr App R 113.
8　Padfield N and Liebling A with Arnold H (2000) *An Exploration of Decision-making at Discretionary Lifer Panels*. Home Office Research Study 213. Home Office, London.
9　Sedgwick J (2001) *Dangerous People with Severe Personality Disorder Initiative Progress Report*. Home Office, London.
10　Lloyd C, Mair G and Hough M (1994) *Explaining Reconviction Rates: a critical analysis*. Home Office, London.
11　Hare R (1991) *The Hare Psychopathy Checklist – Revised*. Multi-Health Systems, Ontario, Canada, p. 3.
12　Hare R, Clark D, Grann M and Thornton D (2000) Psychopathy and the predictive validity of the PCL-R: an international perspective. *Behavioural Sciences and the Law*. 18(5): 623–45.
13　Hart S, Hare R and Forth A (1994) Psychopathy as a risk marker for violence: development and validation of a screening version of the revised psychopathy checklist. In: J Monahan and H Steadman (eds) *Violence and Mental Disorder: developments in risk assessment*. University of Chicago Press, Chicago.
14　Cooke D and Michie C (1999) Psychopathy across cultures: North America and Scotland compared. *Journal of Abnormal Psychology*. 108: 55–68.
15　Her Majesty's Prison Service (2002) *Lifer Manual*. HM Prison Service, London.

16 Williams B (1991) Probation contact with long term prisoners. *Probation Journal.* **38**(1): 4–9.

17 Kemshall H (2001) *Risk Assessment and Management of Known Sexual and Violent Offenders: a review of current issues.* Police Research Series Paper 140. Home Office, London, pp. 21–2.

18 Maguire M, Kemshall H, Noaks L *et al.* (2001) *Risk Management of Sexual and Violent Offenders: the work of Public Protection Panels.* Police Research Series Paper 139. Home Office, London.

19 Bryan T and Doyle P (2003) Developing Multi Agency Public Protection Arrangements. In: A Matravers (ed.) *Sex Offenders in the Community: managing and reducing the risks.* Willan Publishing, Devon.

20 Her Majesty's Inspectorates of Prisons and Probation (2001) *Through the Prison Gate.* Home Office, London.

21 Hood R and Shute S (1998) *Memorandum to HM Chief Inspectors of Prisons and Probation on Parole Board Decisions Relating to Reviews of Mandatory Life Sentence Prisoners.* Unpublished report to the Parole Board.

22 Coker J and Martin J (1985) *Licensed to Live.* Basil Blackwell, Oxford.

Chapter 15

Concluding comments: a humane approach to working with dangerous people

David Jones and Richard Shuker

The benefits of the therapeutic community in prison

The way that we treat our prisoners is a measure of our civilisation. This is, no doubt, a contentious statement and yet, if the people we work with in prisons represent those with the least developed control of their primitive impulses, then the level of violence of our retribution is an indication of our social maturity. It is a curious thing that the population of Grendon Prison has a higher mean PCL-R score – 24 – than high security dispersal prisons – 22[1] – and yet it manages to operate an intense and demanding therapeutic regime and has a lower level of assaults on staff and prisoners, adjudications (discipline charges) and drug use than other prisons of similar security.

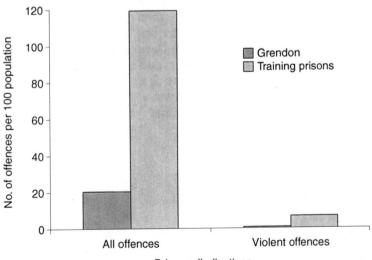

Figure 15.1   Prison adjudications at Grendon compared to closed training prisons

These differences represent real change in the behaviour of inmates as they move from an establishment in the prison estate, or system, to Grendon.

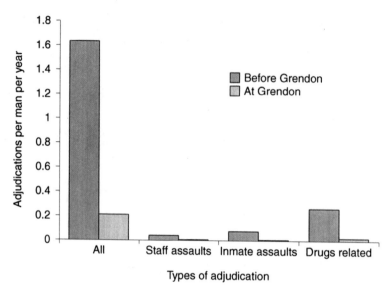

Figure 15.2 Comparison of adjudication rates at Grendon and prior to Grendon

Furthermore, between 50% to 75% of the Grendon group could be identified as having Dangerous and Severe Personality Disorder and were in fact so identified when the original figure of 2500 men was arrived at by the Home Office.

In addition to these clear benefits there have been numerous reconviction studies. These are always difficult to do accurately and require careful matching of control groups. Even when this seems to have been done satisfactorily it can appear, upon further analysis, that this is misleading. For example, a study by Gunn *et al.* in 1978[2] suggested that while there were significant improvements in clinical state there were similar reoffending rates between the two groups. However, post-hoc analysis confirmed that the Grendon men were in many ways more disadvantaged than the comparison group, in having had more illicit drug use and convictions and more alcoholism.[3] Despite these difficulties, on balance there is a reduction in reconviction rates among men who have been to Grendon and this is particularly marked if they have stayed for longer than 18 months.[4]

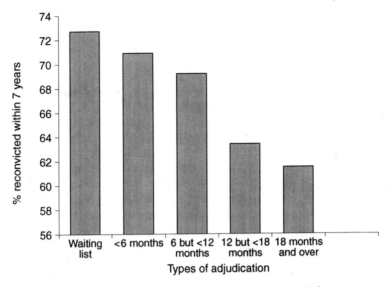

Figure 15.3   Reconviction by length of stay at Grendon (adjusted for risk)[4]

Defining and understanding the therapeutic community

The therapeutic community has provided a treatment structure which integrates social and interpersonal approaches with psychoanalytic psychotherapy. A defining feature has involved attempts to flatten the division between the doctor and patient, recognising the impact of the social structure and context on psychological disorder. This notion emphasises that organisational structure and internal relationships are crucial to an understanding of how a disorder is maintained and addressed.

Therapeutic communities have sometimes been criticised as inaccessible to outside scrutiny and accusations made that they have been reluctant to define and explain their practice. From the other viewpoint, a belief has existed that that any such attempts to quantify their treatment approach within an agreed rationale may only provide an insubstantial and unsatisfactory picture of practice and philosophy.

However, in recent years therapeutic communities have had to define their work in order to retain their credibility and funding both within the health service and the Prison Service.

There are a number of central ideas that characterise therapeutic communities:

- a culture of enquiry: everything – all aspects of community life, all decisions and behaviour – is open to scrutiny and exploration
- the regime is deliberately structured to allow patterns of behaviour to emerge, meaning that . . .
- members' experiences, reactions and behaviours mirror those experienced when outside of the community

- the living learning experience – that is, the idea that every aspect of the regime and members' lives relate to therapy and all situations from the mundane to crisis are used as opportunities for learning.

This particularly applies to interpersonal relationships, where people experience an environment, some of it structured as unstructured, deliberately designed to promote social interaction, and patterns of behaviour emerge in a vivid manner.

These core ideas recognise the importance of:

- allowing problematic or pathological behaviour itself where it provides a means of developing insight and change
- shared responsibility: responsibility for aspects of the day-to-day running of the organisation is taken by residents
- giving decision-making powers to the residents on matters regarding treatment and organisational issues
- social feedback – regarding the immediate impact of behaviour upon others and being held accountable by the community for the wider consequences and implications of their actions.

Therapeutic communities and the 'What Works' agenda

As described in Chapter 5 the predominant doctrine of the correctional and prison services in Great Britain and North America has been the cognitive behavioural approach relating to criminogenic need. So powerful has this lobby been that at one point the terms of reference for accreditation bodies included the clause that treatments (programmes) had to be cognitive behavioural. Thus the question for therapeutic communities has been whether a treatment modality using an approach which has largely focused on aspects of personal distress, neurotic symptomatology and deficits in interpersonal functioning can claim to be able to provide a sufficiently inclusive and specific mode of intervention to tackle offending. There has recently been some shift in this position since it was clearly the case that the Grendon and other therapeutic communities produced good and effective work. The United Kingdom Prison Service now has a distinct accreditation panel for therapeutic communities.

The task has been to describe what happens in therapeutic communities, how it is managed, how staff are trained, how the process is recorded and how change is measured. This is then contained in about 1000 pages of manual, but the difference between this manualisation and the structure around other, cognitive behavioural, programmes is that there is considerable flexibility about what happens in the therapy itself. In other words, the process and progress through therapy are not confined and restricted in any way.

Within the overall therapeutic community approach it is possible to discern three distinct treatment styles.

Psychodynamic

In marked contrast to the cognitive behavioural approach, significant developmental experiences, key attachments, loss and separation are explored. Hearing and trying to understand the individual's history is regarded as of paramount importance. Staff need to be aware of transference reactions as they develop and of their own reactions (countertransference). There is an understanding that the symptom, bad behaviour, will need to acted out (within limits) in order for it to be seen, identified and resolved. These are extremely demanding processes for staff and they need the support of experienced colleagues in order to contain the anxiety and reduce the potential for retaliatory acting out.

Cognitive behavioural

In essence this is a very cognitive behavioural approach to treatment. Interpersonal skills are learned, problem solving and decision making practised on a day to day basis, and boundary keeping and self-management skills emphasised. Members' beliefs are continually explored, behavioural rationalisations examined, and externalisation of responsibility continually focused upon. Perspective taking is learned from the immediate social feedback continually given.

There is a strong behavioural component to this work where an individual behaviour is rigorously examined by other members of the community with surgical precision. As much attention is focused on what triggered and maintained the behaviour as on why the problem exists and why it came into being. Behaviours can be observed and responded to as and when they happen and particular triggers and consequences explored.

Social learning

Likewise, learning occurs through the pro-social culture, where acts of antisocial behaviour such as violence are highly discordant with community values and where the principles of joint problem solving, non-violent conflict resolution and accountability dictate the behaviours which are and are not deemed acceptable.

What happens in the therapeutic community

We now look at the therapy structure and discuss the integration of different treatment approaches within this framework.

A central idea is that all activities relate to treatment. The small groups consist of eight men and usually two facilitators. They meet three times weekly and, while they are generally unstructured, all manner of issues are brought into them. For example, why a particular member had isolated himself during a wing social event or discussions of significant early experiences or an examination of a confrontation between two members took place in a previous session. Especially important is the opportunity for men to learn about themselves from the nature of their own relationships experienced with fellow group members.

The broad content of the group is fed back to the whole community and staff team in a large group immediately after the small groups end.

Full wing meetings, community meetings, are held two times a week, allowing for decision making, voting on particular decisions about community life and discussions about issues of wing conflicts or problems. Staff–inmate relationships are explored, as are problems related to domestic issues, or who has failed to meet education or work commitments.

The treatment groups both inform and are informed by all vocational, educational, work and social activities. In other words anything that happens in the establishment can and often should be fed back into the whole community. Communication is crucial and continuous.

A quarterly assessment is held where objectives are set in collaboration with the group and inmate and progress reviewed. Such objectives are then targets for the therapeutic community to address.

Another important element contributing to the overall success of the therapeutic community approach is that the client member should have a good feeling about the institution. He should be reasonably able to trust the setting that he comes to. There is an element of reality about this; prisoners are used to being tricked, misled and let down. They are used to deprivation. In a therapeutic community the phrase 'it's all grist to the mill' can too easily be an excuse for poor performance or, at worst, sadistic acting out. The institution of the therapeutic community must operate to the highest standards, must have the interests of its clientèle at heart and must be receptive to criticism. Only when those conditions are met can we work effectively with the complex and powerful transference relationships which develop. To fall short of these standards runs the risk of repeating the kind of abuse that many of these men have experienced when children.

The criminogenic agenda

Within this framework the focus on offence-related risk is not seen in isolation from the general personality disturbance but within the context of a treatment approach which addresses both psychological and criminogenic needs.

During the course of treatment an inmate can begin to see links between emotional disturbance and cognitive deficits and the criminogenic factors such as poor coping or interpersonal deficits of relevance to his offending. For example, he can address the deficits in trust and avoidant interpersonal style (which may have been demonstrated during the course of treatment such as in experiencing an anxiety-provoking encounter on the wing), and explore these in relation to the pattern of behaviour (such as maladaptive coping or social isolation) which typified his offending. Likewise he can examine the appraisal biases experienced in treatment where he perceives threat in others, and the chain of events and cognitive processes which lead to his offending.

Offence paralleling

As well as allowing offending behaviour to be seen in the context of general personality disturbance, therapeutic communities also provide a diverse range of opportunities for the assessment of risk and a particular framework for risk assessment as well as treatment.

This leads to the idea of offence-paralleling behaviour, which is understood as establishing links between relapsing behaviour and patterns of behaviour when at liberty. This provides a focus for risk assessment as well as the context for intervention.

The model described here involves developing insight into three areas and identifying links between them as applied to:

- *attachments*: early behaviour, relationships and experiences, domineering/ submissive, trust, empathy
- *behaviour on unit*: for example interpersonal relationships, submissive/ dominant behaviour, passive/aggressive behaviour
- *criminal behaviour*: attitudes to others, interpersonal style, role of fantasy, use of power.

Towards the future

There is clear evidence that a therapeutic community, well organised and well run according to a sound theoretical model, can produce good results with a very difficult client group. The therapeutic community also offers the best model for openness and decency. This can provide the structure and containment for the provision of additional treatment modalities. Although the therapeutic community can be highly cost-effective, it is important not to regard it as a cheap treatment. We shall continue to need the input of good quality, trained staff from a number of disciplines, to maintain the boundaries of the work. It is when these boundaries, around which much of the most potent therapeutic activity takes place, become blurred that standards and effectiveness begin to deteriorate.

Finally, there is a need for further research on the detail of the work in therapeutic communities. Qualitative and comparative studies of the group process and other activities will help us to identify which elements of the intervention are most effective. There is an issue about the treatment of Hare psychopaths, who can be regarded as the most high-risk and difficult-to-work-with group. Reconviction studies will continue to be important and together with careful audit, which takes account of innovative practice, should ensure that high standards are maintained.

References

1   Shine J and Newton M (2000) Damaged, disturbed and dangerous: a profile of receptions to Grendon therapeutic prison 1995–2000. In: *A Compilation of Grendon Research*. HMP Grendon.

2   Gunn J *et al.* (1978) *Psychiatric Aspects of Imprisonment*. Academic Press, London.

3   Taylor PJ (2003) Challenges and successes in forensic psychiatric research. *Criminal Behaviour and Mental Health*. **12**(4): S54–S58.

4   Taylor R (2000) *A Seven Year Reconviction Study of HMP Grendon Therapeutic Community*. Home Office, London.

Index